A Haven in Rathgar

# A HAVEN IN RATHGAR

*St Luke's and the Irish
experience of cancer
1952–2007*

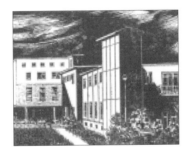

Tony Farmar

A. & A. Farmar

British Library Cataloguing in Publication Data
A CIP catalogue record for this book is available from the British Library

ISBN: 978-1-906353-01-8

First published in 2007
by
A. & A. Farmar Ltd
78 Ranelagh Village, Dublin 6, Ireland
Tel +353-1-496 3625 Fax +353-1-497 0107
Email afarmar@iol.ie
Web www.aafarmar.ie

Editing, design, typesetting and index
by A. & A. Farmar
Cover designed by Kevin Gurry
Printed and bound by ColourBooks

# Contents

# *Acknowledgements*

Writing a history like this is a social process, involving many people. My first thanks go to the members of the History Committee, Derry O'Donovan (Chairman), Dr Michael J. Moriarty, Reggie Redmond, Lorcan Birthistle, Dr John Cooney and David Murnaghan. They commissioned the history and provided constant feedback.

In St Luke's my main and constant contacts were CEO Lorcan Birthistle, Marie Comiskey, Secretary to the Board, and Gay Doyle in the library, without whose joint help I would have got nowhere. Reggie Redmond was tirelessly helpful in several ways, and his history of Oakland (published as Appendix 1) is a real contribution to the local history of the area.

In the course of research I conducted interviews with Lorcan Birthistle, Janette Byrne, Breda Carroll, Dr Peter Daly, Josephine Fitzmaurice, Dr John Healy, Dr Bernadette Herity, Prof. Donal Hollywood, Eileen Maher, Dr Brendan McClean, Lia Mills, David Murnaghan, Dr Michael Moriarty, Derry O'Donovan, Brian Slowey, Phil Sutton, and Padraic White. Written recollections I drew on were by Esther Byrne, Mary Dixon, Eddie Mulligan, Mary O'Loughlin, Kay Rochford and Ted Russell.

Fr Tom Davitt of the Vincentians, Prof. Terence Dolan, John Horgan, Robert Mills of RCPI Library, Dr John A. Murphy, Dr Fred Pfeiffer and Sr Katherine Prendergast of the Daughters of Charity, all provided timely information.

Last but not least I have to thank my partner Anna for putting up with the pre-occupations of yet another medical history and then editing it with such care.

*Tony Farmar*
*November 2007*

# *Chairman's Foreword*

St Luke's Hospital in Rathgar has been serving the needs of cancer patients and their families from every corner of Ireland for more than fifty years.

This is the story—with all its drama—of the evolution of the hospital, of the political and institutional world it inhabited, of the continuous improvements in the treatment of cancer and outcomes for patients and of the remarkable affection in which it is held by patients and their families.

St Luke's has succeeded in achieving a 'double' rare enough in human institutions. It combines technical excellence in the delivery of radiation treatment with an outstanding level of patient care and devotion. It is the major and most specialist centre of radiotherapy in Ireland with an international reputation. It continues to have the loyalty and support of patients and their families who have experienced its services as manifested, for example, by the fundraising initiatives in every parish in Ireland by the Friends of St Luke's.

Now, St Luke's is embarking on another transition as part of the first National Cancer Control Programme with eight designated Specialist Cancer Centres providing treatment for all forms of cancer and delivering diagnostic, surgical, medical and radiation oncology services on the same campus. The hospital is contributing its expertise to the development of this national network and to the migration of radiotherapy to St James's Hospital campus in some seven to eight years. In the meantime, the radiotherapy treatment units (Linacs) at St Luke's are being increased by one-third (from six to eight) and two units replaced thanks to the commitment of €15 million by the Minister for Health, Mary Harney TD.

St Luke's will therefore continue to treat and care for cancer patients for many years to come. We believe that this haven in Rathgar, with its many facilities and tranquil, therapeutic environment, can then support a wide range of complementary care for patients receiving treatment at the Specialist Cancer Centres being developed and we are working jointly with the Friends of St Luke's and former patients to achieve that outcome.

On behalf of the Board, I wish to thank Derry O'Donovan, Chairman of the History Committee, the members Dr Michael J. Moriarty, Reggie Redmond, Lorcan Birthistle, Dr John Cooney and David Murnaghan, the secretary Marie Comiskey, author Tony Farmar who has done a wonderful job in bringing this story to life and CEO Lorcan Birthistle on whose 'watch' this history was conceived and developed.

*Padraic White*
*Chairman*
*November 2007*

# Prologue: Opening the new hospital

For more than fifty years St Luke's Hospital, in the leafy Dublin suburb of Rathgar, has been caring for cancer patients from all over Ireland. Since its formal opening in May 1954 hundreds of thousands of patients and their families have experienced the special care that the hospital and its staff have provided. Some patients have been resident, more have been treated as out-patients. During the course of their treatment, many have established a very close relationship with the hospital.

As the premier facility for dealing with this frightening and isolating disease, the hospital has provided a haven for sufferers. As one patient said recently: 'People feel protected when they enter this hospital and for cancer patients that is a wonderful and welcome feeling and something that cannot be easily replaced. The moment you walk in the door you know that you are in a special place and that you will be looked after.'[1] The carefully preserved landscape with its gardens, old trees and view of the Dublin mountains, and the deliberately fostered lightness and brightness of the buildings add spiritual solace to the physical care provided.

The opening of St Luke's Hospital was a triumph for the not-long-formed Cancer Association of Ireland. This smart modern hospital was to be the focus for Ireland's campaign against cancer. Smart it was, too—architect Thomas Paul Kennedy won the Royal Institute of the Architects of Ireland Gold Medal for aspects of the early design.

The core of the hospital was the handsome house, Oakland,

* *Notes and references start on page 158*

which since 1893 had been the residence of Charles Hely, of the great printing and stationery firm. It had previously been the home of Henry Todd of the well-known department store Todd, Burns. Hely very considerably developed the old house whose origins can be traced back to the 18th century.[2] He built a billiard room (now the Oratory) and extended the wing from the present board room to the Chief Executive's office. He redecorated the dining room (now the board room), the sitting room (the Library) and the drawing room (Clinical Trials Unit) with elaborate silk tapestry and ceilings painted by a specially commissioned Italian artist. These can still be seen. In the grounds he established a croquet lawn, tennis courts, a putting green and ponds, and laid down gardens.

Hely died in 1929, but his widow continued to live in the house. In 1936 she sold part of the grounds together with the avenue from Highfield Road to the present hospital entrance, to which the entrance gates and railings were also moved. Mrs Hely died in 1944, and a few years later her surviving daughter sold the house and lands of Oakland to the Cancer Association of Ireland for £26,000. (This sum is the present-day equivalent of about €500,000, even taking inflation into account, and as such is vividly indicative of the depressed state of the economy and the property market of the day.)

The auctioneers Good and Ganly described the house, in the sedate style of the day, as

> . . . secluded, and yet convenient. Its aspect is south-west and it commands magnificent views of the Dublin mountains. The residence is two-storyed over a lower ground floor. Its exterior is pebble-dashed with granite facings. It has character and charm, and is sufficiently spacious to qualify for the description 'big house' and yet small enough for a family residence. The accommodation comprises, briefly, nine family bedrooms (four of them double) three large reception rooms and some four other rooms on the ground floor; a billiards room, eight servants' bedrooms, kitchens, pantries, and a workroom, as well as accommodation in flats for four gardeners. In addition there is a covered court, rock gardens, fruit gardens, vegetable gardens, tennis courts, croquet lawn, putting green and a wide variety of summer houses and out-houses—all on a secluded, well-wooded site 2½ miles from the centre of Dublin City.[3]

St Luke's was part of an ambitious schedule of government hospital building that was made possible by the continuing flow of income provided by the Hospital Sweepstakes. According to *The Irish Times* over £20 million was earmarked for this, which included £800,000 for a new fever hospital in Clonskeagh, and £1 million each for Galway General Hospital and the Limerick Regional Hospital.

With the death rate from tuberculosis coming down at last, attention was being drawn to cancer, and, as *The Irish Times* noted, 'it is a fact that facilities for treatment of cancer are far from what would be desired. Accordingly, the new cancer service has been encouraged to undertake a far-reaching programme in regard to the provision of hospital facilities, stocks of radium and surgical treatment.'[4] St Luke's was the first and most visible activity of this programme.

Once the land was bought, careful thought went into the planning of the new 160-bed hospital. The architect, Thomas Paul Kennedy, was a specialist in hospitals, working as architect to the Hospitals Commission since the late 1930s. Educated at University College Dublin, he and his friend Gerald McNicholl (later principal architect to the Board of Works) decided to round off their architectural education in 1936 with a two and a half month sightseeing tour of landmarks of international-style architecture in Europe. A highlight of the tour, as he would recount, was when he and McNicholl had somehow found themselves cycling on an autobahn, and were very nearly obliterated as Hitler's motor cavalcade swept furiously by.

Quite soon after completing St Luke's Kennedy became President of the Royal Institute of the Architects of Ireland. Among other hospitals he was involved with was the new Coombe. In his obituary, the *Irish Architect* noted that 'he was one of the most gifted architects of his generation and yet a modest man'.[5]

Great care was taken in establishing the hospital to preserve the natural amenities of the house. One of the first jobs was a detailed survey of the gardens and trees, and during the building no tree was cut down that could possibly be preserved, and all the garden features were specially protected against damage.

The first stage was to convert the old house into a hostel for patients currently undergoing treatment at St Anne's cancer hospital in nearby Ranelagh. The capital's other cancer hospital, in Hume Street, was also invited to send patients, but did not do so. The hostel was complete by May 1951. Then a treatment centre was set up, and this was opened in October 1952 by the Minister for Health, Dr Jim Ryan. It enabled St Luke's to engage in treatment of its own patients and in the first year some 735 new cancer cases were examined and treated.

In May 1954 Dr Ryan returned to St Luke's for the formal opening of the newly-built main hospital building, bringing the accommodation up to 160 beds in all. As Ted Russell, the Chairman of the Cancer Association, noted in his speech, 'this was a welcome addition, as the growing number of patients had for some months overtaxed the existing accommodation.'[6] Dr Ryan performed the opening ceremony, being presented with a gold key by the architect. Then, as *The Irish Times* put it, 'the large party present, including the Lord Mayor of Dublin, Alderman B. Butler, officials of the Corporation, members of the medical profession and business men inspected the hospital.'

St Luke's was open for business.

# Chapter 1: The dread disease

Cancers have afflicted humans for thousands of years. Literary and archaeological records show pharaohs and kings dying from what most probably were cancerous conditions. The disease's very name was bestowed by the legendary Greek doctor Hippocrates, who flourished in the 5th century before Christ. Hippocrates was a contemporary of Plato, and recommended treating breast cancer, but not internal or 'occult' cancers, with surgery. Archaeological remains have identified probable cancers in ancient Peruvian Incas, in Saxon remains in England and in Egyptian mummies. St Peregrine, the patron saint of cancer sufferers, was miraculously cured of a tumour on his leg in 1325. Reaching back in time, a possible malignant tumour (Burkitt's lymphoma) on the jaw bone of a pre-human hominid was discovered in 1932.[1] Stretching further back still, dinosaur remains have been discovered with what appear to be cancerous bone growths and the results of brain tumours.

### Cells—the measure of all things

At the basis of all life is the cell, a tiny citadel of molecular activity that draws nourishment from its surroundings, grows, reproduces and reacts to external stimuli. This basic building block of all life is so small that several thousand can sit on the dot of this i. Cancer is what happens when cells malfunction.

It used to be said that 'man is the measure of all things'. In the widest biological sense this is as wrong as it is to say the sun goes round the earth. In fact, the creatures we can actually see—humans, animals and plants—are really evolutionary exceptions, outliers on the great tree of life. At the centre of this tree, and taking up most of its branches, is the extraordinary dense elaboration of single cell creatures—amoeba, bacteria and a host of more obscure species. It is now estimated that the combined dry weight of these tiny creatures is equal to half the weight of all living organisms on earth. They inhabit every environment from sulphuric acid caves to the frozen tundra.

Small as they seem to us, creatures this size are 'normal' in the sense that by far and away the most numerous living things in the world are single-celled. Recent estimates suggest that there may be as many as 400 *species* in the average human gut. Their importance to our daily comfort is revealed by the simple fact that one of the reasons we often find foreign food difficult is because our stomach bacteria are not used to it.

Plants and animals, including humans, are basically enormous gatherings of cells that cohabit for efficiency's sake. (Generally in nature, the larger the creature, the more efficient the energy usage.) Coming together has enabled the cells to specialise, so there are over 200 different types of cell in the human body. Muscles, nerves, bone, skin—all the organs of the body—are all made of different specialised cell types plus the connective tissue they create. These tissues vary greatly, from the hard and dense, as in bone, to the tough and flexible, as in tendons, to the soft and transparent, as in the jelly of the eye. But all are made of materials extruded from specialised cells, just as a spider extrudes its web.

Of course the coordination of so many cells and cell types requires elaborate systems for cell–cell signalling and for cell–cell cohesion, not to mention specialist functions such as the infection-fighting white blood cells called lymphocytes. Anyone who has tried to organise two teams of five-a-side for a regular knock-up in the park on Saturday afternoon has some glimmering of the complex coordination that has to go into making the trillions of cells in the average human work together so that, for instance, a tennis player can see and return an 80 mph serve. Science is only beginning to unravel some of the ways in which this astonishing phenomenon, human life, operates. Cancer has its source in that complexity.

Many cells, especially those of the skin, the blood and the stomach are so constantly exposed to the stresses and attacks of the outside world that they need to divide and renew themselves very frequently.

As a result, the question 'how old are you?' is not a simple one—the most visible bit of the body, the skin, actually renews itself every two months; stomach cells, in the front line in the struggle with the outside world, every few days. (And if, for any reason, they are prevented from dividing in the normal way, for instance as a by-product of radiation or chemotherapy, the result is nausea, diarrhoea and vomiting.) Even the apparently solid structure of bone is constantly renewing itself, so that it is replaced every ten years or so. The adult human body is not, as it seems, an achieved artefact, like a building, it is a work in progress; we are not aware of it, but every bit, except the brain, is constantly being rebuilt, broken down and rebuilt again.

The human body is thus in constant self-renewing turmoil. Literally millions of cells will have divided in the time it took to read these paragraphs. And with trillions of cells in every human body, dividing and replicating themselves all the time, some every few hours, others over longer periods, the occasional copying mistake slips through the defences. This 'mistake' establishes cells that grow without respect to the numerous checks and balances in the body. Usually this does not matter, either because the growth resulting is benign or because the malign growth is so slow that it is not life-threatening. (And in evolutionary terms it is generally irrelevant, since most cancers occur in those past their procreative stage—nature does not waste effort on quality of life.) Cancer, in fact, is an accidental by-product of life.

### Disease in Ireland

Surprisingly, it is only in the 20th century that cancer has become a prominent public enemy in Ireland. However, every generation before had its reigning disease—one that was feared and hated above all. In the early Middle Ages it was leprosy, still faintly commemorated in Dublin's Leopardstown and, it seems likely, Chapelizod.[2] Then around the 15th and 16th centuries it was plague, a disease so virulent that it seemed at the time that it might wipe out humanity—but then mysteriously disappeared in the 1600s. In the 18th century the disfiguring killer smallpox was feared above others. In the 19th century various 'fevers', notably typhus, the great killer in the Famine years, and cholera, were the prime concern of medical men. In the first half of the 20th century tuberculosis was feared, all the more because it was particularly young men and women that were most affected.

As late as the 19th century cancer was thought of as an uncommon, difficult disease. The great textbook *The Practice of Medicine,* published in 1848, by the internationally renowned Irish medical teacher, Robert Graves, contains only two references to cancer, both underlining its unfamiliarity. People did distinguish generally internal and external cancers, the former being dangerous and uncertain of diagnosis. The outlook for the latter was more cheerful, since they were susceptible to surgery and often—though perhaps they were not real cancers—to quackish treatment by local 'wisemen'. Alarmingly, this is no advance on Hippocrates' ideas of 2,200 years before.

The reason for this lack of medical knowledge was that cancer was regarded as rare. In conjunction with the 1851 Census, Sir William Wilde (Oscar's father) wrote a detailed description of the causes of the 1.3 million Irish deaths in the 1840s.[3] Sir William devotes very little time to cancers: the brief mention includes the fact that the Irish term for the disease is '*Aillsi*", which he translates as 'the foul flesh disease'. The vagueness was typical. As the contemporary Edinburgh specialist Dr J. H. Bennett wrote: 'Medical practitioners are continually in the habit of confounding various kinds of structures and growths under the terms cancerous, or as they call it "malignant".'[4]

The real fear for doctors and lay people in the 19th century was the generic disease called 'fever'. They thought of typhus, cholera, measles and the flu as basically the same. Robert Graves devoted no fewer than 23 out of 70 chapters to 'Fever'. There is a lesson for our time in this. Because this one word tied together trivial ailments with life-threatening ones, any 'fever' seemed dangerous, and the slightest symptom was taken deeply seriously. In the same way, cancer is in fact a hundred or more separate diseases connected by a process. The cancer process works itself out in very different ways depending on its type, just as the feverish inflammation does. Some cancers, for instance non-melanoma skin tumours, are relatively trivial; others, such as advanced lung or pancreas cancers, are very serious. Many doctors believe that a great deal of fear and misery would be alleviated if we took the courage to look the disease more closely in the eye and rid ourselves of the habit of talking just of 'cancer' for this wide range of ailments.[5]

During the hundred years since the Great Famine of the 1840s the living conditions of the Irish people greatly improved—few now lived in the squalid huts that had been common before. As a straightforward consequence most people lived longer. The proportion of the population over 45 years of age rose steadily. And it was noticed that the older the population, the more cancers were experienced. The proportion of the population over 45 years of age was 22 per cent in 1881, and rose to 24 per cent in 1901. By 1936 it had reached 29 per cent. The incidence of cancer rose accordingly. The simple mathematical reason for this is now well understood—that cancers are caused by mutations in the cell, and the more time available the more mutations can be expected.

With the triumphant discoveries of the bacterial origin of so many diseases, medical men in the late 19th century expected that cancer would be found also to have a similar origin. Sir James Paget, the famous surgeon, (described by his pupil Christopher O'Brien, the founder of St Anne's, Ireland's first cancer hospital, as 'a great and lovable man') certainly thought it likely. Since 'in tuberculosis, syphilis, leprosy and the rest there is for each a specific morbid material in the blood, so we should believe that there is at least one in cancer.' Twenty years later the Belfast physician William Whitla in his *Practice of Medicine* cast doubt on the parasite theory but was excited by the recent discovery that mice could be made to suffer from tumours very similar to human ones. He reported enthusiastically on the early use of literally millions of mice in the cause of a cure for cancer.[6]

*Cancer at the beginning of the 20th century*

At the beginning of the 20th century, the Registrar General of the day undertook an extensive survey of the incidence of cancer in

Ireland.[7] He discovered that cancer death rates had risen from 27 per 100,000 population in 1864, the first year of registration, to 65 in 1901. (It is now 190 per 100,000.) This steady upward trend was echoed in England and Wales, where the increase over the same years had been from 39 per 100,000 to 83. Widening the focus, it was clear that this was not just a local phenomenon. Deaths from cancer in the last decade had gone up 30 per cent in Austria, 18 per cent in Holland, 21 per cent in Italy and 17 per cent in Massachusetts.

This was not some worldwide epidemic, but the result of changing health conditions in the developed economies. Better food and living condition (including specifically the removal of animals from living quarters), supplies of clean water, and improved waste control all led to a gradual strengthening of immune systems. As a result, bacterial diseases (such as tuberculosis) only affected the very young, the old and particularly adolescents—those whose immunity was otherwise stressed. Reducing the impact of bacterial disease on the under-45s opened the door for others that affected older people. In the Registrar General's figures for 1904, for instance, 87 per cent of cancer deaths were in the over-45 age category.

His figures revealed that most Irish cancers affected the digestive system, notably the stomach. (Cigarette smoking did not take off in Ireland until the 1930s.) But cancers of the breast and uterus were almost equally prevalent, so there was a well-marked bias towards women dying of cancers. Just as today, different parts of Ireland had different incidences of the disease. In 1909 there was also an east-west split, with rates being considerably higher in the urbanised areas of Dublin and Armagh (85 and 105 deaths per 100,000 respectively) than in Kerry (26) and Clare (38).

The Registrar General asked his general practitioner correspondents, especially those in the high-risk Armagh districts, to identify cause and triggering conditions. A few queried whether the apparent growth in cancers was not a statistical artefact caused by improvements in diagnosis. We have seen how unclear the identification of cancers was only fifty years before. Generally, however, the increase was regarded as real. The answers reveal how far we have since come in understanding the disease.

In his 'Summary of Facts' the Registrar General digested the opinions of his medical correspondents:

(1) That in many cases Cancer recurs in the same family: grandparents, parents and other relatives of the person affected having suffered from that disease.

(2) That frequently where a member of a family is afflicted with cancer, other members of the family suffer from tuberculosis. [He also noted a similar association with (3) epilepsy and lunacy and (4) syphilis.]

(5) That in some instances Cancer has occurred in persons who have been in direct contact with Cancer patients.

(6) That the disease has manifested itself in individuals using the tobacco pipes of persons suffering from Cancer of the Lip.

(7) That in some instances more than one case of Cancer has occurred amongst different families living in the same house or amongst successive occupants of the same house.

(8) That in a few cases the disease has appeared in different houses in the same locality about the same time.

(9) That Cancer not infrequently appears after wounds and injuries.

(10) That in some cases Cancer has supervened where there has been irritation of the lip consequent on smoking clay pipes.

(11) That Cancer frequently shows itself where unfavourable conditions as to residence, food etc. exist.

As practical men, the Registrar General and his medical colleagues assumed (wrongly) that cancer would fit models like other known diseases, and if a 'fit' could be achieved they would then be in a position to propose likely remedies. The 'Summary' shows them trying, for instance in (1) an hereditary model; in (5), (6), (7) they can be seen adducing evidence to fit a contagion model; in (9) a trauma model, in (10) an irritation model, and in (11) a kind of miasma model. Not all of these ideas were completely wrong: there is an hereditary element in some cancers; persistent irritation and other triggers to mutation can be significant. Crucially, however, there was no idea that cancer is a disease of the human cell.

Many of the 20th century's popular fallacies about the causation of cancer can be seen here getting official endorsement from the profession—that it is strongly hereditary; that it is frequently caused by a blow (this was thought to apply especially to breast cancer); that it is caused by some kind of germ; that it is caused by excessive tea, fatty food, damp. However, one long popular idea, that fruits, especially tomatoes, are implicated, was not accepted.

### The first cancer hospital in Ireland

There was one hospital specialising in cancer in Ireland at the beginning of the 20th century. In the City Hospital for Diseases of Skin and Cancer (later St Anne's), which had been founded in 1899, Dr Christopher O'Brien applied the new techniques he had learned on the Continent during his studies in Denmark under Finsen, in France under the Curies and in Germany under Roentgen. He used x-rays and Finsen sun lamps to cure superficial cancers and other skin ailments such as lupus. O'Brien's standing can be judged by the distinguished medical staff, including Sir Francis Cruise, Sir Thomas Myles and Sir Charles Cameron, that he attracted to the work.

Started in Beresford Place by Dr O'Brien with the aid of a group of businessmen, when the hospital moved to Great Brunswick (now Pearse) Street in 1904 it had ten beds and two Finsen lamps, an x-ray machine and a small amount of radium.[8] O'Brien was an enthusiastic user of radium. 'When Radium is judiciously employed,' he wrote in 1924, 'it has no equal in the cure of superficial cancer.'[9] As a digression, it is worth noting how the special nature of cancer had forced medical men to redefine the term 'cure'. The common-sense meaning of 'restore to sound health' was no longer useful in the face of the complexity of cancer. O'Brien defined 'cure' as meaning removal of the tumour followed by six years of remission. He noted with irony the fury that this restricted definition produced; in 1906 he was denounced in Dublin Corporation as fraudulently touting for public money since everyone knew that cancer was incurable.

In 1910 the lease expired and the hospital was forced to close its doors and send the patients home. It is presumably no coincidence that at this time Dr Andrew Charles and another group of businessmen established the similarly named City of Dublin Skin and Cancer

Hospital in Hume Street. However, Dr O'Brien's hospital re-established itself in 1911 in Holles Street (across the road from the maternity hospital).

The connection between skin and cancer in fact was driven more by technology than diagnosis. At the end of the 19th century the new discipline of radiotherapy seemed to be effective for internal and external cancers, and in an age before antibiotics radium and x-rays were applied to the host of chronic inflammatory and non-specific lesions that were at least unsightly, if not also disabling and even dangerous to life. 'Radiation was recommended [in the early days] and widely used in the treatment of pyogenic infections, chronic tuberculous adenitis and the innumerable non-specific conditions that plague the dermatologist and the ophthalmologist.'[10]

The 1920s were a tough time for the managing committees of many voluntary hospitals, as traditional donors left the country or struggled financially. By 1925 the committee running O'Brien's hospital was running out of steam, and decided to hand it over to the French Sisters of Charity of St Vincent de Paul.[11] They soon moved the main hospital to Northbrook Road, keeping a clinic in Holles Street. The nuns renamed the hospital St Anne's, and it was under this name that the hospital was united with St Luke's in 1989.

The move of the hospital to the suburb of Ranelagh was not without controversy. The residents strongly objected to the potential decline in land value caused by the establishment of a skin and cancer hospital in the road. This classic not-in-my-back-yard response perhaps also reflected more visceral fears. There was a widespread belief that cancer was somehow contagious; and lacking close medical attention many patients would have allowed tumours and skin infections to develop to a distressing extent. Court proceedings were initiated, but unfortunately for the residents the ground lease, while prohibiting 'offensive' or 'noisy' trades could not be stretched to prohibiting a hospital. Although protests continued, the hospital stayed in Northbrook Road for more than fifty years, and is now a clinic.

O'Brien retired in 1927, but before that he had left a record of his ideas about 'The Cancer problem' as he saw it.[12] He was not optimistic. In terms of understanding the disease, he wrote, 'we stand today where the ancients stood, baffled and bewildered by darkness and impenetrable gloom, despite the millions spent on cancer research.' O'Brien identified three current theories of cancer. The first was the so-called 'constitutional theory', which held that cancer was the result of 'an inherited disposition'. The second was the 'irritation theory' by which any repeated mechanical irritation 'permanently alters the mechanism of cell-division and ultimately produces cancer'. Clay pipes, soot irritation and jagged teeth were all adduced in favour of this idea. The third theory was the micro-parasitical one mentioned above. A strong argument in favour of this theory was the prevalence of stomach cancers, then one of the most prominent types. The President of the London College of Surgeons believed in this so wholeheartedly that, as he put it, 'for many years I have avoided eating all sorts of uncooked vegetables. Much as I enjoy salad with my chicken or my cheese, I do not touch it.'[13]

By this time the rate of death from cancers had reached 100 per 100,000 and was rising to meet that of the rapidly reducing tuberculosis rate. In 1928 the Registrar General commented in his *Annual Report* on the trend:

> The continuous rise in mortality from cancer is one of the outstanding features demonstrated by vital statistics, especially in recent years, when this disease has assumed an important place among the causes of death. The increase has not been continuous from year to year, but successive rises indicate the advance that is being made by the disease. This is particularly the case since 1923.[14]

Sometime in the mid-1940s the death rate from cancer overtook that from TB, and it has been rising steadily since.

### (Not) talking about cancer

The way we feel about a disease reflects and is reflected by literature and ordinary usages. A small number of diseases—such as fever, leprosy, plague and few others—are so seared in the brain that they are regularly used as public images. Cancer is one of these, whereas tuberculosis is not. On the other hand, in the 19th century tuberculosis certainly established a literary niche as the disease of the sensitive,

hectic, artistic, oversexed and doomed. Thomas Mann characterised one of the patients in his sanatorium as 'laughter-loving Marusja
with the little ruby on her charming hand, the handkerchief with
the orange scent, and the swelling bosom, tainted within'.[15] The
'delicacy', as it was also called, had an almost glamorous reputation.
(This was before the far from glamorous *Mycobacteria tuberculosis*
had been identified as the cause.)

Cancer would never become remotely attractive. It was no more
than 'the loathsome canker [that] lives in the sweetest bud'.[16] It was
also a word and an idea that people feared and felt the power of—
they do even now.

The public debates in the Dáil and Seanad show this in action.
There were a mere 31 uses of the word 'cancer' in the twenty years of
Oireachtas debates up to 1940, compared to 258 occasions when the
word 'tuberculosis' was used. Most of the uses were technical or in
the context of medical research. A few deputies used the word as a
metaphor, revealing much about how people thought of cancer at
the time. In the 1922 Treaty Debate Michael Collins memorably
referred to the struggle against the 'slow steady economic encroach
by England . . . the cancer that was eating up our lives'.[17] This reference was taken up by Professor Hayes of the National University of
Ireland who referred to 'another cancer even more important, eating into the very heart and vitals of the Irish nation, the spiritual
penetration, the sway of English manners and customs, of the English tongue, English ideas and English ideals in Ireland.'

Later, in the 1930s, unemployment is referred to as a cancer, and
in 1936, somewhat unflatteringly, in the course of a debate on parti-
tion, Deputy Hales referred to Irish nationalists as potential 'cancers
capable of eating into the heart of the British Empire'.[18] Cancer is
frighteningly portrayed as a silent, sinister, unstoppable, undermin-
ing growth—malignancy personified. How deep this implacable
image went, and how different it made the idea of cancer can be
appreciated if one contemplates the idea of referring, for instance,
to the smallpox of unemployment.

The 'Big C' was characterised in people's minds as a painful
death warrant. (In County Cavan cancer was referred to as 'The

Lad',[19] in much the same spirit as the Greeks referred to the terrifying Furies as 'The Kindly Ones.') It was, as one author noted

> . . . the most emotive disease of modern times. The very word strikes fear and despondency into the bravest heart, and for many people the diagnosis of cancer is synonymous with a sentence of death. Seen as a form of malign invasion from without by a foreign entity, which is gnawing away at their vitals and over which they have absolutely no control, cancer has become associated with an inevitable progress towards a painful and degrading death.[20]

The slow humiliation of gathering weakness and the probability of extreme, unstoppable pain were part of the dread. For the devout majority in Ireland there was also the psychological terror of God's judgement (the result of which no one could be certain) and the associated fear of purgatory or an eternity in hellfire.

### Treating cancer

Part of the fear of cancer arose from the fact that by the time the patient presented symptoms to the doctor it was likely to be too late to do anything. In 1941 Dr Oliver Chance, then Medical Director of St Anne's and later to become the first Medical Director of St Luke's, reported that some 60 per cent of cervical cancer patients reported to him for radiotherapy at St Anne's were classified as stage III or stage IV.[21] Perhaps this was part of the reason why his five-year survival results were markedly worse than those from the Holt Radium Institute in Manchester or the Madame Curie Hospital in London. He himself put the difference down to the fact that the work in those two great specialist hospitals 'is carried out by a large and expert staff of gynaecologists, radiologists, physicists, laboratory workers, etc. working as a team in a properly equipped hospital.' Women's lives would be needlessly sacrificed, he concluded 'until a similar hospital is set up in Ireland.'

In 1936, the Hospitals Commission (the committee officially charged with allocating the extraordinary flow of income derived from the Hospitals Sweepstake) took up this point in its *First Report*, an examination of the Irish hospital system. Cancer, it found, was

> . . . the third single cause of death (apart from senility), tuberculosis

being the second. Whilst the mortality from the latter disease is steadily decreasing, due in part at least to the measures taken by the State 30 years ago, that from cancer is steadily increasing and the time cannot be long when it will occupy the second place in the Cause of Death statistics.[22]

The Commission identified just two hospitals devoted to cancer—St Anne's, Northbrook Road, and the City of Dublin Skin and Cancer Hospital in Hume Street. They were both in Dublin. By the 1930s, however, there was little reason for continuing the technology-driven combination of skin and cancer diseases, as both hospitals still did. (In the early 1920s Hume Street had declared itself also specialist in kidney disorders.) The *Report* commented that it was 'difficult to see a connection between skin diseases and cancer . . . the treatment of cancer is almost exclusively confined to surgeons and radiotherapists, while that of skin diseases falls mainly within the domain of the physician'.[23]

By 1936 St Anne's had 83 beds of which just about half were usually occupied. Hume Street was smaller than St Anne's, with 48 beds. It was governed by a carefully balanced group of six Protestant and six Catholic trustees and conducted by a medical superintendent, Dr Andrew Charles. In 1931 this hospital had been the subject of a vehement debate in the Oireachtas, which suggested that all was not well. The occasion was a Seanad debate about whether Hume Street should receive Sweepstake moneys. Senator Oliver St John Gogarty, an ear, nose and throat specialist, vehemently objected, describing the hospital as a 'one-man show' and an 'attempt to make a corner in cancer in Ireland.' Damningly, he went on to describe the hospital in Hume Street as 'a cancer farm', and as such superfluous and unnecessary. Gogarty was certainly inclined to flights of rhetoric, but his comments were supported by the great elder statesman of Irish medicine Sir Edward Coey Bigger, and by one of the members of the Hospitals Commission.[24]

In practice, the bulk of cancer patients were treated in the general hospitals, either by surgery, or in the few better-equipped places by surgery and radiation treatment. In official medicine in Ireland by the 1930s these were the two possible routes to a cure—from the patient's point of view providing a choice between the obvious violence of surgery or the alarming new science of radiotherapy. (Chemotherapy was not to appear on the scene for many years.) More or less radical surgery was attempted in a large proportion of cases, with often doubtful quality of life for the survivors. The need to eradicate all the cancerous cells at once drove surgeons to a 'better safe than sorry' policy, and cutting away substantial parts of the patient's body. The second route was radiotherapy, which also had a major palliative use in reducing tumours if not actually curing the patients.

Outside official medicine there was, as usual, a vigorous flora of quack medicine, though cancer cures were much less widely promoted than those for TB. In country areas 'wisemen', like the farmer Johnny Sweeney of Athlone, would provide cures for external cancers (or what were reputed such). His cure, wrote May Green, 'used herbs, egg yolks, dandelions and cow dung, but that was not the whole secret. He mixed the ingredients in the holy water of the old church.'[25] And if all else failed, there was divine intervention to pray for. The national pilgrimage to Lourdes always contained a high proportion of those with tumours and malignancies, and many came back strengthened spiritually if not physically. More mysterious were the numerous holy wells and holy bushes throughout the country, relics of pre-Christian theologies.

Although all hospitals treated cancer patients, at the time of the 1936 *Report*, apart from St Anne's and Hume Street, only St Vincent's, the Mater and two other of the twelve general hospitals in Dublin (St Kevin's and Baggot Street) had equipment for anything more than diagnostic x-ray work. It was clear to the Commission therefore that

> . . . the fight against cancer has hitherto been carried on in a more or less desultory fashion. For this, financial stringency has been largely if not wholly responsible. The prevention, diagnosis and treatment of cancer have not been approached from a national point of view, individual hospitals and individual medical men making what limited provision their financial resources allowed.

The Commission was of the opinion that the tremendous cost

of the new radium and deep x-ray treatments made it 'apparent that any rational system of cancer treatment will require centralisation'. This had been done with success in Sweden, the first country in the world to establish a central institute for the treatment of cancer.

Pressure to this end came also from the largest source of radium in the country, the radium committee of the Royal Dublin Society. Leading the drive was the seventy-year-old Sir Edward Coey Bigger, whose most public moment had been his 1917 *Carnegie Report* on the physical welfare of mothers and children in Ireland, in which he highlighted the problem of infant mortality by declaring that it was more dangerous to be a new-born baby in Dublin than a soldier in the trenches.

Although by the mid-1930s most hospitals had a diagnostic x-ray department, therapeutic use of x-rays was limited to a few large hospitals, and radium was used even less. Two of the pioneers in its usage, Maurice Hayes and Walter Stevenson, had died in 1930 and 1931 respectively, and thereafter the usage of the supply kept by the Irish Radium Institute (based in the RDS) had dwindled to less than a quarter of the potential.

In 1933 Sir Edward visited British radium centres in an attempt to see how usage might be increased in Ireland. He conservatively estimated that there were then about 3,000 cancer cases in Ireland, but 'very few of these persons are being treated with radium. The chief reason is that there are very few medical men with the necessary knowledge and training to carry out the treatment.' Money, which hopefully would be forthcoming from the Sweep, was needed to establish proper training and technical facilities.[26] The Hospitals Commission entirely agreed. They followed up their *First Report* in December 1936 with another specifically recommending a centralised radio-therapeutic institute on the Swedish lines. They also proposed that a cancer council be established to act as the governing body of the institute and 'to direct a well organised campaign against cancer in the country, to co-ordinate the activities of all hospitals, surgeons and radio-therapeutics.'[27]

The Minister snapped into action, and by mid-1938 the Provisional Cancer Council was established. The chairman was Dr Patrick

MacCarvill (a dermatologist from St Anne's with an impressive record in the War of Independence) and among the fourteen members were Dr Oliver Chance, Professor Barniville from UCD and Sir Edward Coey Bigger representing the RDS, as the premier organisation in the country holding radium at the time. Unfortunately, the Council had barely time to sort out its expenses and establish an office (complete with fourteen Chippendale-style chairs in Rexine and a brass plate) before the Second World War broke out.[28] In the new conditions international travel was obviously out of the question, and getting information from hospitals was not going to be easy. Furthermore, the potential source of finance dried up as postal censorships imposed across the world put a stop to the international sale of Sweep tickets. Dependant on sales only from Ireland, the Hospitals Commission's income dwindled to a mere 3 per cent of the pre-war level. The great offices of the Hospitals Trust in Ballsbridge were let out to the Department of Supply for the duration.[29] In May 1940 the Council's activities were formally suspended and the files were mothballed.

The consequence was that just as the number of Irish people dying from cancers exceeded those dying from tuberculosis for the first time, the slight effort there had been to create a coordinated national approach to cancer was put to gather dust in the back offices of the Department of Local Government and Public Health.

# Chapter 2: Burning rays

We have seen that the Hospitals Commission in the 1930s called for a central radio-therapeutic institute for Ireland along Scandinavian lines. The key reason for establishing a centralised service was the simple practical fact that treatment plants using the powerful new medical tool of radiation from x-rays and radium were unprecedentedly expensive to establish and to run.

## *The burning rays*

There were two sources of the so-called ionising radiation—that is, radiation with enough energy to remove electrons from atoms inside the cell, for good or evil. These mysterious burning 'rays' at the centre of the new medical science were first created artificially and called 'x-rays' in 1895. A few years later, initially Becquerel and then Marie and Pierre Curie identified natural radiation, originally in uranium, then in the new mineral polonium (named after Marie Curie's native country) and finally in the much more energetic radium in 1898. The basic principles of x-rays discovered all those years ago are still at the heart of the sophisticated new computer-guided radiotherapy machines in St Luke's today.

Wilhem Roentgen of the University of Wurzburg had discovered in 1895 that if a high-voltage electrical current was passed through a vacuum the fast-moving electrons colliding against a metal plate produced rays which clouded a photographic plate.[1] Experimentation very quickly revealed that these rays were not easily stopped by paper, wood or even light metal, nor by soft human tissue. However, materials with a higher atomic number (lots of protons and electrons etc.) such as metal and, crucially, the calcium in bones, would stop more of the energy. As a result, the photographic plate or film would show dark where most of the rays had gone through soft tissue, and light where they had been absorbed by bone. A skilled eye could detect subtle but medically significant variations in the absorption rates.

The new discovery attracted instant attention among scientific men here. It is said that the first x-rays in Ireland were taken in 1896 by Rev. Henry Gill of Clongowes, or possibly by a Monsignor Molloy of Maynooth.[2] However that may be, it is certain that by March 1896 Professor Barrett of the Royal College of Science in Dublin had produced the first clinical x-ray in Ireland, revealing the whereabouts of a broken needle in a girl's hand. Dr William Haughton installed an x-ray apparatus in Sir Patrick Dun's in that same month, thus becoming the first practising radiologist in Ireland. Haughton remained for many years a prolific writer on radiological topics.

The ability of x-rays to penetrate the soft tissues of the body and to reveal the bony structure underneath was an immediate public sensation. A new medical world seemed to be opening both for diagnosis and for therapy as the rays provided a clean and effective alternative to the knife. And in a world where personal modesty was so highly valued, the x-ray's ability to penetrate previously hidden parts of the body was both exciting and alarming. Jokes were made about how the new rays could spot eavesdropping servants, and women feared intrusion. It is said that one sharp entrepreneur successfully produced a line of x-ray proof underwear.

At the same time the Curies in Paris had begun to explore the complex force fields of the nucleus of the atom. They were especially interested in those unstable elements now called radioactive (a term they coined). Like a sailor tossing excess baggage overboard until the keel sits evenly, these continually emit dangerous particles until an energy-efficient and stable state is achieved. When enough of the radioactive material has gone through this the original source effectively becomes harmless. These emitted particles are called alpha and beta radiation and gamma rays. For our purposes gamma rays, which are the same type of radiation as x-rays, are the most important. The only difference between the two is that one comes from a high voltage source and the other is a natural product of radioactive decay.

Gamma rays have numerous separate effects on cells, including on the cell membrane, on the oxidative processes, on growth and cell death triggers, on protein triggers used in communication with other cells and, critically, on the DNA repair and recombination process in the nucleus.[3] This ability to kill tumour cells was the crucial addition to the medical armoury against cancer.

The apparatus used in radiotherapy produces ionising radiation by two different methods. X-rays of varying energy intensity can be produced by high voltages—the higher the voltage the more energetic and penetrating the x-rays. The second source is the natural emission of gamma radiation from radioactive sources.

The deadliness of ionising radiation derives from various phenomena. First, the energy delivered may simply kill the cell. If enough are killed, this interrupts a crucial bodily housekeeping function. We have seen how frequently in a healthy adult cells constantly die and need to be replaced. If too many are killed, for instance as a result of exposure to ionising radiation, the replacement rate drops drastically and vulnerable bodily functions cease to be performed, like a football team which mysteriously loses a third of its players.

Second, the power of ionising radiation to affect electrons and so molecules can cause various problems inside the cell, most notably genetic mutations. These disrupt the complex chemical pathways inside the cell, so that, for instance, defensive quality control signals are ignored, or perhaps the external signals which govern when a cell should divide and so grow and when it should not. Part of this message specifies what kind of special function the body as a whole requires the cell to perform. This message is usually damaged in tumours. As a result tumour cells are relatively unspecialised. One reason that radiotherapy works against cancer is because relatively primitive tumour cells, with their different internal chemistry, are more easily damaged than healthy cells. With care, it is possible to kill the malignant cells but leave unaffected the more differentiated cells which surround the tumour.

Although the original focus of 'medical electricians', as they were called, was on diagnostic use of x-rays, the therapeutic uses soon became apparent. It seemed as if nature had presented us with a combination of a really powerful sun-lamp, and, used in a different way, a radiation knife. The first cures of cancer patients were reported in 1899; these were all skin or superficial tumours, for it was not until the 1920s that x-rays could penetrate to more deeply seated cancers.[4] Dr Rankin of the Royal Victoria Hospital in Belfast was an early pioneer, publishing an important paper in 1906 on the 'Treatment of malignant disease by x-rays'.

It took some time for researchers to discover the full power of the new rays—one famous story tells of the painful burns that Becquerel suffered as a result of carrying around a phial of radium in his waistcoat pocket. More tragically, many of the early researchers suffered serious lesions, especially to their hands, and many died of leukaemia and diseases such as the aplastic anaemia which killed Marie Curie. The first Medical Director of St Luke's, Dr Oliver Chance, was believed to have had no fingerprints as a result of handling radium needles.[5]

An early method of measuring the dose of radiation delivered by primitive machines was to test the dose against the operator's skin. If the skin reddened, the so-called erythema dose had been achieved. But of course the reddening of the skin was symptomatic of damage to the operator's cells. For many years pioneers such as Walter Stevenson of Dr Steevens' Hospital, who, with Professor John Joly of Trinity College, invented the technique of using radium needles in the treatment of cancer, struggled with unreliable x-ray equipment and uncertain outcomes. In the early days, for instance, the quality of vacuum tubes used in the x-ray equipment was such that as a session progressed the tube would get hotter and the nature of the x-rays change. Quite soon, however, the critical importance and difficulty of delivering the right dose only to the malignant cells, sometimes deep inside the body, with as little as possible damage to the healthy ones, was realised.

The technology only allowed the radiotherapist to deliver a box-shaped 'hit' of radiation. The trick was to ensure that the tumour, whose likely shape was much more irregular (more like a fist than a brick) was encompassed in that box, with a safety margin. Obviously that meant that healthy cells were going to be affected, and the objective was to expose as few of them as possible. As it happens, recent research stresses that tumours are not separate from the body, as it were like a marble on a plate. They are more like a member of the family with some vicious habits but who still lives at home. A constant flow of molecular messages passes between all cells; this happens also between apparently healthy cells near the tumour and the cells in the tumour itself. The so-called 'tumour-associated host cells' are thought to be implicated in the growth processes of the tumour and so it may in fact be just as well that the radiation process attacks them as well as the actual tumour cells.

As time went on it became clear that tumours were not made up of an undifferentiated mass of a single type of cell, but were heterogeneous like ordinary tissues. Radiation affects these types more or less lethally, so that a dose which effectively kills some cells leaves others unaffected. This obviously has implications for dose planning.

### The new Department of Health

In 1947 the government finally established an independent Department of Health. The unit had previously been a subsection of the Department of Local Government and Public Health. Ireland was, in fact, one of the last countries in Europe to have a stand-alone Department of Health, no doubt largely because of the vehement opposition to 'socialised medicine', as they called it, from the medical profession, from the Boards of the hospitals and from the Catholic Church hierarchy.

The standpoints of these three groups were different, but each was to cause problems in different ways for the grand idea of a national cancer centre. The medical profession had been skirmishing against the state since the beginning of the century, when they tried to resist the obligation to report certain infectious diseases, claiming that it was the householder's responsibility. In every such discussion, the doctors' most often expressed fear was that they would lose their much-prized professional and financial independence. They hated the idea, as they often said, of sinking to becoming mere state employees—like the civil servants they were so often negotiating with. Professor R. A. Q. O'Meara, later the key figure in a joint research venture between St Luke's and Trinity College, characterised this prospect in a lecture to Trinity students in 1955. The new doctor, he declared gloomily, 'will have to resign himself to a future in which others will select him as a suitable cog to replace one which is outworn, in a machine from which there is no escape.'[6]

The Boards of the hospitals (many of whose members were doctors) simply disliked the idea that their establishments, into which so much devotion had been poured, would be interfered with. A particular source of resentment was the hi-jacking, as they saw it, of the income from the Sweep by the Department. From their point of view, Sweep tickets were sold on the basis of support for Irish hospitals; consequently all the income should come directly to the hospitals. This argument would have been stronger if there had been any cooperation at all between the various hospitals in their development activities. This did not stop doctors' leaders from talking casually of the treachery of the Department and 'the blind avarice of the state' when discussing such issues.[7]

The third key group, the Catholic Church, combined a visceral fear of communism with devotion to the doctrine of subsidiarity. This principle of Catholic social teaching, as enunciated by Pius XI in his encyclical *Quadragesimo Anno* (1931), stated that it was 'gravely wrong' for a higher organisation to take over duties that could be performed by a lower.[8] The doctrine certainly provided a useful barrier against totalitarianism in Mussolini's Italy. In the Irish health service, however, a measure of centralisation was precisely what was needed. The rule of subsidiarity meant that if a family or a hospital could provide (pay for) medical services, the state should not attempt to do so. The implications for all sorts of state-directed medical provision, not just the later Mother and Child scheme, were obvious. Following the Pope's teaching, Archbishop McQuaid regarded such provision as 'an injustice and at the same time a grave evil and disturbance of right order', and so resisted it across the health service.

# Burning rays

## *Introducing DNA*

At the heart of the complexity of the human body lie cells, and at the heart of cells lie the immensely long strings of DNA which drive everything. Cancer is a result of malfunctioning DNA. Surprisingly, it is quite recently, certainly within the working lifetimes of the St Luke's senior consultants, that this has been enunciated. The structure of DNA itself was only revealed in 1953, a year after St Luke's first opened. And the two scientists responsible, Francis Crick and James Watson, have both reported their indebtedness in this epochal achievement to an event that had occurred ten years before in, of all places, wartime Dublin.

The date was February 1943, just at the turning point of the Second World War. By extraordinary heroism the Russians had inflicted on the German army their first defeat in the Battle of Stalingrad. In Dublin the physicist Erwin Schrodinger, who would win the Nobel Prize for physics in 1993, presented his ideas about the fundamental factors affecting the transmission of life to a bemused audience in Trinity College. At this time Schrodinger was in exile from his native Germany because of his objection to the race laws, and was happily housed in de Valera's Institute for Advanced Studies.

The lectures, as James Watson put it, 'elegantly propounded the belief that genes were the key components of living cells and that, to understand what life is, we must understand how genes act.'[9]

The lectures were published a year later under the title *What is life?* The importance of Schrodinger's speculations, combining quantum physics with biology, can hardly be overestimated. They defined and focused the thinking of a whole generation of molecular biologists, not least Francis Crick and James Watson. This led to the central scientific achievement of the late 20th century, the explosion in understanding of the mechanisms of cells, the essential pathway to understanding cancer.

At the time, of course, Schrodinger's exposition was barely understood, and certainly not by *The Irish Times'* reporter, who, obviously far out of his depth, attempted to turn one of the lectures into a sensational attack on the dangers of x-rays. 'Detrimental mutations—or in plain language deficiencies—in the gene or hereditary treasure of living organisms' will be caused by x-rays, he reported. These were 'passed on to the offspring, and several generations later may become harmful'.[10] Perhaps the reporter should have stuck to stories such as that carried on 6 February about the woman of a hundred-and-one from County Wicklow, who vividly remembered the Famine, and did not disapprove of smoking or make-up, but thought that lipstick was an invention of the devil.

### Towards a national cancer service

In the meantime, wheels had been put in motion once again to establish a coordinated national cancer service in Ireland. In 1944 Dr James Deeny, a general practitioner from a well-established Catholic family in Lurgan, had been appointed Chief Medical Adviser to the Department of Local Government and Public Health. He immediately set about making waves. Although, as it happened, he was no friend of St Luke's, a facility that he thought 'it was a mistake to build',[11] his energy and drive were to be the key factors in the evolution of the Irish health system for the next fifteen years, and this, of course, included the cancer service.

Quite soon after his arrival in the stately Custom House office of the Department he did a study of cancer deaths for the ten years 1936 to 1945.[12] He noted various shifts in the incidence of cancer, for instance to fewer stomach and mouth cancers, the former unexplained, the latter probably due to better mouth hygiene and better dentistry (fewer ill-fitting, chafing dentures, he guessed). Skin cancers of the face and neck were also reduced, which he attributed to an improvement in the employment conditions of fishermen, horse carriage drivers and ploughmen.

His discussion shows that the medical profession had advanced considerably in its understanding of cancer since O'Brien's 1924 article. 'The distribution of the disease,' Deeny wrote, 'shows that cells which exist throughout their life in the internal media of the body, maintained at correct temperature and pH and with constant chemical equilibrium of the surrounding body fluids, do not often show cancerous changes. Whereas those cells subject to either varying physical and chemical influences or to prolonged external irritations are more readily affected.' He was groping towards the insight that it is the busy, front-line, and therefore frequently-renewing cells that are most likely to become cancerous. The more often cells renew themselves by dividing, the more opportunities there are for cancer-creating errors in the reproduction of DNA. In the absence of pollutants such as cigarette smoke, the most frequently replaced cells are just the ones that most often become cancerous.

Deeny noted the slow, steady increase in the number of cancer deaths over the previous thirty years, pointing out that the very steadiness of the trend proved that this was not an epidemic phenomenon, but was caused by underlying factors. He ascribed it largely to the increasing number of susceptible persons as the population aged, and perhaps partly to improved diagnostic skills. At the time of writing he believed that 'almost 60 per cent of cancer deaths [were] due to gastro-intestinal cancer', but there was a marked increase in the incidence of cancer of the lung, up from 48 deaths in 1936 to 133 in 1945 (still, however, a small proportion of the total of just under 4,000 cancer deaths per year). No connection with cigarette smoking was made, for Richard Doll's path-breaking epidemiological studies of smoking and cancer were a few years in the future.

Following up this research, in May 1947 Deeny wrote a Departmental paper proposing that a new committee be established to advise on the development of the country's anti-cancer services.[13] The key to such a service, as he saw it, was the radiological facilities, whose primary function would be to reveal the early stages of cancers. The first aim of the service would therefore be to provide technical assistance so that the whole country would be covered by adequate diagnostic x-ray facilities.

In the early 1950s Deeny was to organise the mass radiography service which provided exactly such facilities for tuberculosis, and was a major contribution to the eventual elimination of that disease. Unfortunately, he did not understand that cancer is not really one disease but many, with growth habits and outcomes as varied as so many different plants in a garden. Consequently, the kind of one-shot solution that worked so well with tuberculosis would not work with cancer.

The next stage, Deeny proposed, was to establish a (small) cancer institute for curative treatment, preferably in the grounds of St Kevin's (now St James's) Hospital. A cancer hospital outside the city would provide accommodation comparable to sanatorium pavilion blocks for long-stay patients.

The Minister, Dr James Ryan, accepted the general thrust of Deeny's proposal, and in January 1948 invitations went out to Dr Patrick MacCarvill, who had been chairman of the Provisional Cancer Council, and others, inviting them to sit on the proposed Consultative Cancer Council. Among the members were Dr Oliver Chance, then of St Anne's, later the first Medical Director of St Luke's; Finbarr Cross, later of St Luke's; State Pathologist John McGrath of Trinity, who, it was said, had 'figured in most of the murder trials of the previous twenty-five years'; M. J. Brady, a deep x-ray and radium specialist from Hume Street; and the distinguished Trinity physicist E. T. S. Walton, who was to be awarded a Nobel Prize in 1951 for his work on nuclear physics.

The new Council's first meeting was in April 1948, by which time there had been a change of government, and the new Minister, Noel Browne, seized the opportunity to tell the press how urgent the cancer problem was. At the same press conference the chairman Dr Patrick MacCarvill rejoiced that the Council was so bluntly named:

> There is nothing to be gained by suppressing the name 'cancer'. On the contrary, a more frequent use of the term will, as in the case of tuberculosis, help the public to realise that there is no stigma attached to it, that it is not necessarily a harbinger of death—rather that it is something for which if aid is sought in time much can be accomplished. In many of its forms it can be completely cured. Many lives can be saved, life can be prolonged in comparative comfort and the disease deprived of its painful associations.[14]

After foreign consultation, notably with the Christie Hospital in Manchester and the allied Holt Radium Institute, which were to become models for St Luke's, the Consultative Cancer Council issued its report in July 1949. Its key recommendation, moving away from what James Deeny had proposed, was that there be a single body 'under whose control all activities in connection with the [cancer] service be carried out.'[15] In the absence of figures of incidence (as opposed to mortality) they estimated that the cancer service should cater for some 6,000 cases a year, and warned that this was likely to rise (though it is unlikely they had any idea of the present 20,000 cases a year).

### Radiation treatment in the 1950s

By the time the Consultative Cancer Council delivered its report in July 1949 the basic principles of radiotherapy had been defined. Although, as one contemporary author wrote, 'the nature of the action of the ionising radiation upon living cells [was] still obscure',[16] there were by then numerous techniques for delivering ionising radiation to tumours. The voltage used to produce increasingly penetrating x-rays had crept up to 140 kV in 1913, 200 kV in 1920 and 300 in 1925. The 250 kV x-ray cannons or deep x-ray machines would become the work-horses of St Luke's. Typical treatments involved a filtered dose at intervals over several days or weeks; the rays generated could penetrate about 10 centimetres into the body. The next substantial advance in x-ray technology came in the 1960s, with the development of megavoltage linear particle accelerators.

These treatments were delivered as an external beam, as were those using 'radium bombs', so called from the fancied resemblance of an early version to a Mills bomb used in the First World War trenches. In the 1950s radium bombs began to be replaced by the cheaper and more powerful cobalt-60 bombs.

Complications arose because each tumour is subtly different in shape and size, and it is also a living part of the body, so it moves and alters shape with everyday activities. In planning the dose, issues such as beam direction (entrance point and target), the number of beams, the likelihood of affecting critical structures near the tumour, the likelihood of permanent damage to skin and other tissues, whether to deliver the desired dose in a few or many repetitions all had to be considered, often with quite small amounts of information to go on. A key consideration in the search for higher energy machines was that the way these machines delivered the radioactive dose spared more of the healthy tissue overlying the tumour.

Radium was also the basis for a series of techniques in which the sealed radioactive source is placed very close to the tumour. One of these brachytherapy ('near to') techniques was pioneered by Walter Stevenson of Dr Steevens' Hospital, who substituted numerous radium-filled serum needles around the tumour for a single source placed on the skin above the centre of the tumour. Other treatments used radium needles embedded into the tumour, radium sources placed inside the body or sources placed on a material (radium mould) a few millimetres from the skin's surface.

### The new cancer centre

The immediate practical question for the Department of Health in the late 1940s was how 'the provision, staffing, equipment, administration and maintenance of a radio-therapeutic institution' (as the brief to the Provisional Cancer Council had put it) was to be organised. The cost and elaborate staffing requirements of the new plant were problems that the Irish health service had not previously encountered. Up to then medical equipment had been a minor charge. The Hospitals Commission analysis showed that surgery and drug costs amounted to less than 15 per cent of the costs of running 29 general hospitals in 1933. This new equipment was not only expensive to purchase, but since it required highly specialised staff it seemed expensive to run and maintain. Apart from the cost of the equipment (which in effect meant that a single central institution was the only practical route), significant practical and operational problems could be envisaged.

The novelty of the problem perhaps induced the Consultative Council to take an over-optimistic view of the organisational task. They proposed in their report the establishment of a single Central Cancer Board with three radio-therapeutic and surgery centres, in Dublin, Cork and Galway. Immediately on its establishment the Central Cancer Board was to take charge of a pool of the beds, personnel and specialised equipment presently allotted to cancer by the two skin and cancer hospitals. They did not think that either of the existing Dublin hospitals was capable of suitable expansion, so, as quickly as possible, a 'modern centre equipped with full facilities for radio-therapeutic and surgical work, and comprising all necessary departments for the ancillary services and research' was to be built.

This was to be a substantial new hospital, with 160 beds, intended to provide radiotherapy and surgical cancer services for as much as two-thirds of the Irish population. The magic figure of 60 cancer beds per million population, derived from Scandinavian experience, was much touted. 'Existing facilities in Dublin,' the Council proposed in their report to the Minister, 'will be concentrated in the newly-built centre, and a suitable use found for such existing hospitals as will have the major part of their work transferred to the new centre.' Blithely, the Council suggested that 'with good will on the part of the hospitals, and a reasonable approach by the Board, no insuperable difficulties will arise.' After all, as they naively wrote: 'All concerned are sure to appreciate that the claims of cancer sufferers for immediate attention in an improved service outweigh all other considerations.' Unfortunately, a recognition that some restructuring is in the patients' interests has never been sufficient to effect change in the Irish medical service.

The practical problem posed by the high technology plant seems to have misled this experienced group of men into believing that a benign outcome was likely.[17] A bit more realism entered into their discussion of the familiar surgical services for cancer. Although the Council believed that 'if cancer surgery could be centrally concentrated . . . the surgeons specialising in different branches of cancer surgery would become more perfect in technique with an improvement in results not otherwise to be achieved', they had no hope that this would happen. It was 'not considered a practical proposition'— which was a coded way of accepting the insuperable obstacles presented by vested interests.

Within weeks of receiving this report Noel Browne had opened discussions with the veteran politician William T. Cosgrave with a view to his becoming Chairman of 'a body to establish a proper cancer service' to be called the Cancer Association.[18] Cosgrave, the first President (as the office of Taoiseach was then called) of the Irish Free State, and since 1932 Leader of the Opposition, had not long retired from politics. He was an interesting choice; however, although he was initially keen, the idea came to nothing, perhaps because Browne rejected a proposal of Cosgrave's for membership of the Board. It is unlikely that they found each other politically congenial.

So Browne turned to a colleague in Clann na Poblachta, Limerick businessman Ted Russell, who had stood for the Dáil as a Clann na Poblachta candidate in 1948 and was to stand again in 1951, both times unsuccessfully. Russell, educated like Browne at an English public school, was then in his mid-thirties. He came from an old Parnellite family in Limerick and was for many years chairman of his family milling and provender business. He finally sat as an Independent TD from 1957 to 1961, before retiring to local politics, having already been Mayor of Limerick in 1954. Although he knew nothing of cancer before he took on the job, Russell settled down with enthusiasm to what he later called his 'most significant contribution' to public life. There does not seem to be any doubt that Browne specifically told Russell that he should have a free hand in developing the cancer service.[19]

The new Cancer Association held its first meeting in November 1949, in Leinster House, with Noel Browne in attendance; also present were the seven proposed directors, headed by Ted Russell and the Secretary of the Association, solicitor Liam Egan. In 1950 a series of quick decisions showed that the new Association meant business: in January members travelled to the Christie Hospital and Holt Radium Institute in Manchester; it was agreed to set up a cancer centre in Cork; in February it was agreed that the operation of the Dublin cancer centre should be through a single unit (and that any rail travel undertaken by Board members should be at first-class rates).[20]

Negotiations were established with the existing hospitals, St Anne's and Hume Street, but it very quickly became obvious that for different reasons neither would cooperate in the larger scheme. Then it was proposed that land behind the existing St Anne's Hospital in Northbrook Road be the site for a greatly expanded hospital there. Board member Oliver Chance, who was on the staff of St Anne's, approached the Sisters for their opinion. They referred the query to Fr J. P. Sheedy, the head of the British and Irish province of the Vincentians. His response (copied to Archbishop McQuaid) made it clear that the Sisters would not sell St Anne's, that they were unable to lease the hospital to the Cancer Association and they were not willing to become employees of the Cancer Association either in St Anne's or elsewhere. [21] When later the Minister sought to nominate members to the board of the proposed enlarged St Anne's, the Archbishop refused, expressing his complete confidence in the ability of the Sisters to manage the hospital. In view of the large expenditure that would be required to complete the expansion, the Minister did not feel justified in continuing without state representatives on the board. [22] In a later letter to Archbishop Dalton of Armagh, Dr McQuaid elaborated: 'The position is grossly unsatisfactory, in that a monopoly is being created that will crush our two voluntary hospitals.[23]

After this rebuff, and a less blunt one from Hume Street, who proffered, as the saying goes, 'every assistance short of actual help', the Cancer Association decided in May 1950 to advertise for a green-field site. In June they took on their first employee, clerk-typist Maureen McElroy. Then somebody spotted that a large house in Rathgar called Oakland, with 13 acres, was for sale.

Things moved quickly. At a special Board meeting the Secretary was authorised to bid up to £36,500 for the house and grounds, and, including all fees, spent £29,000.[24] It is said that the Dublin Jewish community were the under-bidders. Ironically Archbishop McQuaid had given the state cancer hospital, soon to be called St Luke's, another boost by preventing the Rathgar Redemptorists from purchasing the Oakland site. A few days after this purchase, on 29 June 1950, following prolonged negotiations between the Cancer Association and the Department, the Association was formally in-corporated as a company limited by guarantee. Among the directors listed are Russell, T. J. Brady from the Department, Oliver Chance, Patrick MacCarvill, and R. E. Whelan.

Browne had chosen the quick and straightforward form of a limited company, perhaps, as the Mother and Child row gathered heat, being loath to go to the Dáil with the more usual statutory form. An internal Departmental memo written some years later noted that the Association was given 'a wide range of authority and responsibility with the minimum of Ministerial or official control'.[25] However, this lack of statutory status (which Russell and his colleagues, rather simplistically, equated with freedom from bureaucratic control) was long a source of grievance inside the Association.

From the beginning the question of their independence of Departmental oversight was a sore point. As the Association started to spend money, more or less insistent demands from the Department for budgets and plans were increasingly seen as so much interference.

In September 1950 the firm of Kennedy and O'Toole were appointed architects to the Association, and told to prepare plans for a 150-bed hospital. Advertisements for staff began to appear, signalling their ambitions by seeking employees with foreign language skills. A few months later, in February 1951, Dr Oliver Chance resigned from the Board and was appointed Medical Director (at a salary of £2,750 per annum). He was the first of an exodus to the new hospital from St Anne's, including Dr Michael O'Halloran, the second Medical Director, and the Chief Physicist John O'Connor. This loss of senior staff was keenly felt in St Anne's. In an unpublished history of St Anne's the anonymous author commented dryly: 'St Luke, though a doctor, had evidently acquired the art of the fisherman, too.'[26] Quite soon May Dixon, the first Matron, and three trained nurses joined from the Meath, as did the Meath's head porter, Jimmy Butler.

By this time the old house on the site, Oakland itself, had been transformed into a hostel to accommodate ambulatory patients undergoing treatment in St Anne's (Hume Street was offered the same facility but did not take it up). Beds for 36 patients were established in a series of small wards, the largest holding 7. Patients were ferried to and from St Anne's by taxi, accompanied by a nurse. When in the hostel they had access to the grounds, a splendid billiard room (the billiard table was later sold for 100 guineas) and a reading room. Three wireless sets provided for 'listening-in'.

### The Department takes a hand

Meanwhile, the conflict with the Department about the Cancer Association's assumption of independence simmered quietly. In May 1951 the Secretary wrote to the Association pointing out that he had been asking for budgets and plans since 1949; he did not think it was good enough to be curtly told that a contract had just been signed with Cramptons, the builders. 'The Association will appreciate,' he wrote silkily, 'that, in view of the Minister's general responsibility for the health services, it is desirable that he should have at his disposal information in regard to the projected development of the cancer service . . . the value of this report would be considerably enhanced if it were accompanied by a financial statement.' This suave epistle was eventually responded to, in August, by a seven-page report on the Association's activities to date.

Perhaps the Departmental Secretary turned first to the finance section, where the report's author, presumably Secretary Liam Egan, recorded that the Association had received since 2 December 1949 £74,231 of income, virtually all from the Hospitals Trust Board. Costs were as follows:

| | |
|---|---|
| Purchase and refurbishment of Oakland | £33,913 |
| Expenditure on hospital building to date | £13,843 |
| Purchase of radium | £8,737 |
| Purchase of land in Cork | £6,274 |
| Furbishing and equipping a 36-bed hostel | £5,556 |
| Wages, salaries and running expenses | £5,286 |
| *Total expenditure* | *£73,895* |

The Secretary went on to note that the current estimate for completing the hospital was £468,900, a figure that was to be handsomely exceeded. He also enclosed an estimate for the proposed Cork cancer centre of £200,000. This sum brought a sharp response from the Department: 'The estimate given for the Cork Centre is regarded as excessive . . . the Minister therefore urges a radical reduction in the total cost of the project.' £100,000 was regarded as a reasonable sum.[27] Ted Russell and fellow board member R. E. Whelan smoothed this over by a rapid visit to the Minister, James Ryan, but it was a straw in the wind. Next, hackles in the Association were raised by an unexpected visit by the official Local Government Auditor to Oakland where, according to Russell, he demanded that books be produced 'forthwith' and 'directed' that certain insurance be effected.

Another long letter from the Minister attempted to calm things, but the Association's core point, that such audit was neither necessary nor legally justified, was not conceded. In March the following year the Minister sent the Local Government Auditor in again. Russell protested vigorously against what he described as a surreptitious 'attempt to establish dual control' and what he undiplomatically called 'unnecessary bureaucratic interference which can serve no useful purpose except to discourage the voluntary efforts of public-minded men'.[28] He threatened to 'consider his position', though this was clearly bluff. References to the Minister's predecessor were unlikely to appeal, since Dr Ryan was not only of a different party, but also a considerably more practical politician than Noel Browne. This was not a battle the Association could win in the long run. However, they continued, as we shall see in the next chapter, to fight against what they saw as reneging on the promise of the original appointing Minister.

Behind this shadow-boxing, the real work of the Cancer Association, the building of the hospital and the treatment of patients, was going on. Over 700 patients were treated in the first year of operation, and in February 1954 the completed wards were handed over by the architects (together with a bill for a total of £650,000). In May the Minister, James Ryan, formally opened the hospital. It had been, as the *Irish Architect* commented, many years later, 'a building designed and built outside customary Departmental systems and in a remarkably short time by hospital standards'.[29] With the hospital now complete, and the wards full of patients, the Cancer Association entered a new, but hardly less strenuous, phase of existence.

# Chapter 3: A national aspiration thwarted

By the end of the 1950s Ted Russell and his colleagues of the Cancer Association had achieved much. They had started in 1949 with a letter from the Secretary of the Department of Health to Russell which drew attention to two specific objectives.[1] First, 'the provision in Dublin of a modern centre with accommodation for 150-160 beds'—this had been done. By 1957 a newly-built award-winning hospital nestled in the quiet suburb of Rathgar, catering for thousands of cancer sufferers from all over the country. The second objective, to provide a modern centre in Dublin and to ensure that duplication of services was avoided, was to prove more troublesome.

*The new hospital*

St Luke's Hospital was now the major centre for radiotherapy in the country. There was also a surgical unit performing some 1,500 operations a year. The hospital provided both deep and contact x-ray therapy, and was in negotiation with the department for the supply of a so-called 'cobalt bomb' which would provide a high-energy penetrating ray for deep-seated tumours. There were five x-ray therapy units, fully staffed by radiographers. Radium therapy and radioactive isotopes were also in active use. Finally, there were diagnostic x-ray facilities and two operating theatres. The radiation treatments were summarised in a contemporary document as follows, which gives a clear picture of some typical regimes:

> *Breasts* P. op. therapy course usually 20 D.X.T. (4 weeks). City patients can attend as out-patients.
> *C. C. U. or C. B. U.* Usually radium insertions as in-patients (1 or 2) followed by 20-30 D. X. T. City patients can come as O. P. some

only have radium insertions

*Throat* 25-30 D. X. T. Usually confined to bed

*Brain* Usually about 30 D. X. T. Usually confined to bed,

*Palliative treatments* to relieve pain can be any no.

*Cancer of skin* 1-5 C. X. T. City patients as O.P.

*Cancer of lip* Radium implants are usually in Hospital 10-14 days or C. X. T. 1-3 treatments.[2]

Because the public view was that a diagnosis of cancer was equivalent to a death sentence, new patients' first encounter with St Luke's could often be a lonely and frightening event. There was a kind of holy dread about the place itself. The hospital staff were well aware of this, and did their best to counter the fear such feelings inevitably stimulated. The foyer, described in the brochure written to commemorate the launch of the hospital in 1954, was a 'pleasant entrance hall designed to put [the patient] at ease immediately on his introduction to the hospital. Having given the necessary personal details at the reception desk, he passes into the spacious main waiting hall, strikingly handsome and original in design.'

Many of the patients, coming up perhaps from the country, were deeply self-conscious about the deadly, not-to-be-spoken-about disease they were carrying. 'The cosy circle of seats are conducive to friendliness and prevent anyone from feeling alone. As he waits his turn to be called for his first clinical examination the patient may obtain a cup of tea from the nearby buffet.'

This first examination would be made in the fully equipped consultation rooms off the hall. Blood tests were carried out in the laboratory nearby. Once a treatment had been recommended patients were given a further appointment to come in either as out-patients or, if they lived too far away, to take their place in the wards. The work of the hospital revolved round the regular clinics. Ten of these were radiotherapy clinics under the direction of the radiotherapy staff, six were so-called 'combined' clinics, where patients were seen by specialists in surgery, plastic surgery, dentistry, gynaecology, otolaryngology and general medicine and a consultant radiologist. In addition, patients with problem cases requiring radiation were seen at a special daily clinic attended by available radiotherapy staff.

Although most patients attended on an out-patient basis, the

160 beds were also used, there being at least 100 patients resident at any one time. Statistics showed that they typically spent just over a fortnight in the hospital. There were four wards, two on the ground floor and two on the first floor. In the manner of the day, a careful hierarchy distinguished private, semi-private and public wards. Thus, on the ground floor were the male wards, public and semi-private, and also beds for those sad cases of infant tumours. These were under the control of Ward Sisters O'Shea and Lawlor, backed by Staff nurses Brady and Hayes (the stiff formal style, using surnames only, is characteristic). On the first floor were the female wards (with an overspill in the hostel), plus 14 private rooms and the female semi-private. Ward Sisters Coleman and Twomey looked after these wards, seconded by Staff Nurses Gardner and O'Regan.

Although many patients were subsidised by local authorities, very few paid nothing at all. The 1956/7 *Annual Report* notes that the average payment was just £20 per patient, with a mere 10 patients out of 2,400 making no personal contribution. For those choosing to go private, the charges could mount up: a private room cost 10 guineas per week, deep therapy 1 guinea per treatment (which would usually be 20 or more), consultation fee with Dr Chance 3 guineas; if an operation was called for there would be the surgeon's fee plus as much as 8 guineas for the anaesthetist and the use of the theatre.[3] For a private patient, therefore, a stay in St Luke's was unlikely to cost less than 50 guineas. At this time the average industrial wage was about £375 per annum (which is equivalent to no more than €8,000 in today's money).

From the beginning St Luke's acted as the hub of a country-wide cancer service. By 1957 there were clinics in Cork, Waterford, Limerick, Tralee and Castlebar. In that year there were just under 10,000 attendances at these various clinics. Indeed, the success of the clinics established by the Cancer Association had, in the words of a Department of Health memo 'threatened, quite unmistakably, the existence of the other two Cancer Hospitals. St Anne's has reacted by establishing clinics also and we now have the situation that in Galway, for instance, or Castlebar and Ballina, clinics are held by staffs travelling out from both hospitals.'[4]

St Luke's was termed a 'tertiary referral centre', which meant that the patients had typically progressed from the initial diagnosis by the GP to consultation with a specialist who would, if appropriate, refer him or her on to St Luke's to take advantage of the sophisticated services available there. The Cancer Association reported (in 1957) treating patients from all 26 counties of the Republic, including 292 from Donegal, 212 from Kerry, 250 from Roscommon and 129 from Waterford. The bulk were looked after in St Luke's itself, with 7,336 in 1957. (Dr Michael Moriarty, now consultant radiologist, who joined St Luke's in the 1960s, vividly remembers these men sitting up in the wards with their caps firmly on their heads.)

The world that these patients were entering was friendly, if by our customs rather formal. Mary O'Loughlin, a radiation therapist in the 1960s, recalls the hospital being a small specialised place where everyone knew each other. But as she remembers: 'The familiarity of first names was non-existent. Dr Chance was always referred to as "Doctor" as were all the doctors, while others were addressed as Mr, Mrs, or Miss or Nurse.' The formality extended to the annual staff dinner. Once a year at Christmas time everyone was summoned by a printed invitation to gather, in formal dress, in the out-patients' department for sherry. At 8 pm they went on to the dinner. After dinner people were invited to do a party piece, and every year Professor Eamon de Valera, the gynaecologist, contributed 'Molly Malone', with everyone being expected to join in the chorus—so when in the late 1960s Michael Moriarty and other young doctors came to the party they struck a cheerfully different note with the pop song 'Lily the Pink'—'It went down a treat, of course, being such a change from "Molly Malone".' As has been said before, the sixties started late in Ireland.

The second objective highlighted by the Secretary of the Department of Health in his letter of 1949, was 'to ensure by definite and clear agreement with the authorities at present providing facilities for the diagnosis and treatment of malignant diseases that duplication of the cancer service and unnecessary expenditure will be avoided'. This part of the brief proved much more difficult, for there was little cooperation from the two other Dublin cancer special hospitals, Hume Street and St Anne's, and there was very little expectation that the general hospitals would transfer their cancer patients to St Luke's.

There was also a third objective, an important part of the Consultative Council's recommendations, that is 'the development of a comprehensive and coordinated National Cancer Service covering the State as a whole.'[5] It is no doubt significant that this was not even mentioned in the Secretary's letter, though it remained a key aspiration for the Board—for them, St Luke's was only the beginning.

### Ireland in the 1950s

It is difficult, in the affluent 21st century, to think back to the very different days of the 1950s. The population was barely three million, and Ireland was the only European country whose population was actually shrinking. There was not much money, and the moral climate was strongly authoritarian; as a result many people lived sadly cramped lives both materially and personally. As the novelist John McGahern put it, people's first allegiance was not to 'Ireland' but to 'small intense communities which often varied greatly in spirit and character over the course of a few miles . . . in that country individual thought and speech were discouraged. Its moral climate can be glimpsed in the warning catch-phrases: "*a shut mouth catches no flies, think what you say, but don't say what you think*".'[6] For an increasing proportion the escape was to emigrate, and to hope for better lives in the United States or Britain. Young women in particular rejected the lives that their mothers had been offered. Of those who stayed, an extraordinary proportion of both sexes remained single (the Census reported that Irish people had the lowest marriage rate in the world).

The politicians, most of whose attitudes had been formed during the national struggle more than thirty years before, had no solution to the problem of the people leaving the country. Indeed, as Alec Newman, Editor of *The Irish Times*, commented: 'The suggestion is commonplace that it is the natural destiny of the Irish people to emigrate, and our sensible course would be to let the population run down to two millions'.[7] And to be honest, the electorate did not expect much from their leaders—in 1957 they elected Fianna Fáil to power once again, and de Valera, in his 75th year, took office for the tenth time.

Many people, and not only in towns, lived in large family groups in what we would today regard as intolerably crowded conditions. The 1946 Census had revealed that one in ten of the population, over 300,000 people across the state, lived six or more people in houses with three rooms or fewer. Not only were they crowded, but basic domestic facilities were often primitive. Fewer than one-quarter of houses had indoor flush toilets; only one in six had a fixed bath with running water. In these circumstances, the comforts of privacy and cleanliness were not easily obtained. The complacency of the officials and politicians was demonstrated by the description of these results in an official publication as 'a marked improvement in the general housing conditions'.[8]

The decade had started with depressing statements from the Central Bank ('existing standards of living cannot be maintained') and Minister for Finance Seán MacEntee ('the nation is living beyond its means . . . it must spend less'). What they meant was that imports were nearly double exports, and at least half of exports were either live cattle or food and drink, the simplest and least profitable forms of industry. After nearly thirty years of tariff protection Irish business people had adapted only too well to their protective cocoon. A group of American business experts invited by Seán Lemass to report on the Irish business scene in the early 1950s was appalled at the almost complete lack of initiative or entrepreneurial drive they discovered. There was, they sadly remarked, 'no sign of the wild Irishman' to be found.

The expectation of life at birth for men was 64 years, and for women 67 years (it is now 75 and 80 respectively). This average was low mainly because, before the advent of antibiotics, one in ten of all deaths were of children under ten years old. However, the grip of the infectious diseases that were the great killers of the past was being loosened by antibiotics, and now heart disease and cancer, the diseases of age and civilisation, took the greater toll. Of the

36,700 deaths in 1955 nearly 13 per cent were from cancer, and half of those were from stomach cancers.[9]

To look after the sick there were 3,000 registered medical practitioners and 8,400 trained nurses. (There are now, for a population 1 million larger, over 120,000 men and women employed in the healthcare system, including more than 30,000 nurses.) Income from the Sweep (which was mainly spent on hospitals and not, for instance, on community medicine or developing GP services) meant that Ireland had more hospitals per capita than most Western countries. For historic (i.e. largely sectarian) reasons, there were three medical schools in Dublin and six in the country as a whole; there were eleven general hospitals in Dublin alone, not to mention three obstetric hospitals and no fewer than three hospitals specialising in cancer. As Oliver Chance, Medical Director of St Luke's, declared at one meeting: 'Until this position has been rationalised, money will continue to be wasted and the teaching of medicine cannot be efficient.'[10] Running such a clumsy and wasteful system in a country struggling to pay its way was not easy, but proposals to rationalise were quickly silenced by well-connected social and political forces.

Although cancers of all sorts continued to take their toll, the medical sensation of the 1950s was polio. This strange and feared disease was to have its last outbreak in Cork in 1956/7, just as the Salk vaccine was coming on stream in the United States. The reaction to the disease throws vivid light on Irish people's attitude to disease in general, and by implication focuses on cancer's place in the disease spectrum. At the same time the triumphant success of the enormous scientific and medical push against polio had important repercussions on the way cancer research was to be addressed.

Polio, like cancer, had been endemic since at least the time of the pharaohs, and continued to strike from time to time—perhaps the most famous name associated with the disease before US President Franklin D. Roosevelt[11] was the novelist Sir Walter Scott—but it had become widespread in the 20th century, with a dramatic outbreak in New York in 1916 when 12,000 children were paralysed. Epidemiologists noted that it was richer countries such as Denmark, Sweden and New Zealand where the worst outbreaks occurred.

Because public health was improving, especially in better water and sewage systems, the immunity that had previously been part of growing up was no longer able to protect the children. Polio attacks the nerve cells that control muscular movement; paradoxically it was not a disease of the squalor and dirt that decades of medical propaganda had warned against, but of nice, clean middle-class homes.

So when the last outbreak in the western world occurred in Cork in 1956, it was the new suburbs that were worst affected. Over 500 children were permanently damaged in the outbreak. But because only 1 per cent of people who get the disease are seriously affected—most suffer no more than a bout of nausea, sore throat, headaches and perhaps an unusual tingling in the fingers—it is suspected that as many as two-thirds of the 75,000 people in Cork may have been infected by the time the outbreak had run its course in early 1957.

The public reaction was extraordinary. Fear of infection imprisoned people at home. Cork city was deserted; shops, hotels and pubs were empty, to the extent that commercial interests began to put pressure on the *Cork Examiner* to tone down the recording of the outbreak. As the journalist Claud Cockburn was told by a cab-driver: 'The people are afraid. They are afraid to come into Cork. If this epidemic goes on half the shops in [St Patrick] street will be bankrupt.'[12] As the news spread to Dublin, there was panicky talk of isolating Cork and Cork people, of preventing them from travelling to Dublin. One woman wrote a furious letter to the Department of Health complaining bitterly of the irresponsibility of the Department in allowing Cork people to come to Dublin to attend the All-Ireland final, thus putting herself and her children at risk. Hearing a Cork accent, people in public transport moved away from the speaker; in Cork itself houses with known victims were shunned. Seeing a child with the tell-tale callipers supporting his legs, people moved away from him as if he was still infectious.[13]

The very suddenness and aggressiveness of epidemic polio (hitting, as we have seen, as many as two-thirds of the 'target' population) was in itself terrifying. The slow deadliness of cancer evoked dread and fear, but not a sense of the potential treachery of everyday contact. Other factors differentiated the diseases: polio struck the vulnerable young, whom we were supposed to be protecting, ('I'm *especially* fond of children' as the sinister characterisation in a US fund-raising film put it). Cancer, on the other hand, generally affected the older generation, who, to put it into the most callous evolutionary terms, had had their chances. It lacked the poignancy and sadness of the child-crusher, polio.

Polio has been described as 'before AIDS, the disease which most terrified people'.[14] Given the widespread dread of cancer, to the extent that people resisted even saying the word out loud, this may seem difficult to justify. However, cancer, though a much more significant killer than polio, never provoked panic. From time to time ideas were expressed that cancer was contagious, but these were usually batted down by the medical profession. Talk of 'cancer families' and 'cancer villages' was equally discouraged, though when reading of families in which successive generations had died of the disease, it was difficult for the ordinary reader not to believe in some such mechanism.

### *The grim lottery*

In general, cancer was thought of as a kind of grim lottery. It was understood to be a slow, internally generated malignancy, not to be caught from public exposure like a viral disease. If it appeared, one was expected to endure with as much fortitude as possible the inevitable outcome. 'A long and serious illness, bravely borne' was the typically euphemistic death notice. In part because it so often (especially in women) appeared in 'private' parts of the body, it was also a matter not widely to be talked about. Indeed, it was in the strict sense a taboo subject—as Freud describes it, with connotations that are 'awesome' and 'above the ordinary' but also 'dangerous', 'unclean' and 'uncanny'.[15] Thus, typically, 'Our Medical Advisor' writing in the woman's magazine *Model Housekeeping* around this time advises that any lump in the breast should be surgically removed, saying that 'if it is benign, no harm is done, but if it is more serious, treatment may be commenced.'[16] Everyone knew exactly what he meant by 'more serious', but preferred that he did not write the word.

Although it was certainly uncomfortable to read about, there was good information available (as far as the progress of science would allow). In the very last issue of *The Bell* (December 1954), readers were told, accurately enough, that the efficient survival of the body requires that cells of the body regularly die and are replaced, one cell for one cell, by new cells. 'It sometimes happens, however, that certain cells "break the law" and begin to multiply, far exceeding the requirements for replacement. These "extra" cells constitute a group which is called a tumour.'

The professional publication *Cancer* (1957) was able to add numerous incidents of how this 'sometimes happens', adducing the enormous amount of work that had been done in infecting mice and other laboratory animals with potential and actual carcinogens. But in the end the author had to admit that the central mystery was far from penetrated. He could hardly decide, for instance, 'whether tumours usually grow from a single cell or from a number of single cells that have undergone malignant transformation due to a common cause.'[17] Although the mechanism of DNA replication had been exposed in 1953, the significance of the discovery had obviously not penetrated into medical research. The author (a man who had been researching carcinogenesis for twenty-five years) comments: 'The idea of cells having a stage in their activities at which their guard is momentarily down is attractive. Such cells', he notes, 'might represent only a small minority of the local cell population in one instant.' But he goes no further. DNA is not mentioned in the whole 40-page article.

The silence tells us much about the enormous advance in understanding the mechanism of cancer since then. As a recent author confirmed: 'As late as the 1970s, human cancer remained a black box. Theories were abundant: cancer was hypothesized to result from defective immunity, viruses, dysregulated differentiation, mutations'.[18] As is usual in medicine, a rich diversity of theories implies weak or little actual knowledge.

But why did certain cells 'break the law'? Basically no one knew. Current theories in the 1950s, as reported to Dublin's intelligentsia in *The Bell*, proposed that 'cancer [may result] from a malady which occurs during the embryonic period and which develops through survival of embryonic cells during birth; a bacterial or virus infection; of a manifestation of somatic mutation . . . ultra-violet rays have given rise to cancers of the epithelial tissue . . . a number of chemical substances may stimulate the development of cancer'. 'Minor burns, irritations caused by badly fitting dentures etc.', however, are definitely ruled out, as are ideas that cancer is infectious or that 'certain streets or houses are responsible for cancer'.

When his wife was diagnosed in the 1960s with breast cancer, the publisher Seán Feehan wrote: 'Why should mankind's greatest brains have failed to find a cure? Everything so far has been just hit and miss; and it has been mostly miss. Today the word "cancer" is almost synonymous with the word "death".'[19] Because of this, the normal strategy of the day was to keep the patient in the dark about the progress of the cancer. Doctors might give the full details (as far as they thought appropriate[20]) to next of kin, but it was felt that if the patient knew all they might be tempted to 'give up', and cease to 'fight' the disease. (The persistent idea that the psychological attitude of the patient can affect the outcome is traceable back to the beginnings of Western medicine, in the writings of Hippocrates.) In his *Memoir* John McGahern recalls that his mother, in the 1940s, 'suspects that the cancer may have returned, but everyone around her conspires to drive her from this knowledge. Her stomach pains and recurrent bouts of constipation and diarrhoea, she is told, are an unrelated sickness that she can recover from if only she will make the effort.'[21]

*Relations with the Department of Health worsen*

Unfortunately, as the day-to-day routines of the hospital settled down, and the number of patients began to increase, behind the scenes the relations with the Department of Health were coming to a head. After nearly ten years' hard work Russell and his colleagues on the Board, notably R. E. Whelan, a Dublin businessmen, had established both a modern hospital specialising in cancer, and cancer clinics across the country. But the dream of a single central national centre for cancer had eluded them. This was partly because neither St Anne's nor Hume Street, the other two hospitals specialising in cancer, wished for a moment to abandon their independence; nor at the same time did the general hospitals, which provided surgical and other treatment for perhaps half of all cancer patients, propose to hand over this stream of business. As usual in the planning of the Irish medical service, the power of intense local loyalties both of staff and patients, built up perhaps by generations of work and caring, completely swamped the larger picture.[22]

One must suspect also that there was not much enthusiasm from the Department of Health. It was pre-occupied firstly with the anti-tuberculosis programme. An enormous amount of work had been done in respect to this, and with new drugs it looked as if the effort was about to conclude successfully. Then there was the politically attractive building programme made possible by the Sweep—as Dr Deeny recorded, 'in the years 1940–65 more than 200 hospitals were built and another large number reconstructed'.[23] Attempting to force the unwilling into participating in a national cancer centre of excellence was not a high priority. As we have seen, Deeny himself, as the Department's Chief Medical Advisor, was even unenthusiastic about the viability of a stand-alone cancer facility.[24]

The battle-ground of the dispute was the constant wish of the Cancer Association to be left alone to achieve its mandate; against this was the demand of the Department, as the accountable authority under the various Acts, that it control and channel all medical expenditure. The Board of the Cancer Association, the governing authority of the hospital, took the view that a former Minister for Health (Noel Browne) had promised them independence of action, and this they were determined to exercise. As a result they continually interpreted the Department's routine requests for accountability as mere red-tape and interference. Chairman Ted Russell was quoted as saying on one occasion to the Minister that 'the Cancer Association was competent to run its own affairs, and should not be pestered continually with enquiries relating to expenditure.'[25]

Behind Browne's promise and the Board's persistence was a widespread distrust of the civil service. One senior surgeon expressed the commonly held view that 'the dead hand of State control is responsible for much of our difficulties in the teaching hospitals'.[26] This was partly a general suspicion common in the 1950s of centralised state power, which, as the Church never ceased to preach and many believed, quickly led to communism. (Though in truth it would be difficult to imagine a country *less* likely to re-enact the October Revolution of 1917 than de Valera's Ireland.)

There was also a belief in business and medical circles (the origins of the members of the Association's Board) that the so-called 'faceless civil servants' knew nothing of business or healthcare, and the less they intervened the better. In hindsight, it does not appear that either of these sectors had made such a notable success of their affairs. Irish business, as we have seen, was a negligible force. It was also common knowledge that despite large subsidies from the Sweep the great teaching hospitals of Dublin were 'drifting into a more and more alarming financial situation' and the medical service was, as one senior surgeon bluntly put it at the time, 'by no means the best in the world'.[27]

The relationship between the professional and business classes and the civil service was made worse by an undercurrent of class antipathy. The typical civil servant was a bright Christian Brothers boy who had worked hard to get into the service and defeated scores of competitors for the slot. The grandees of the medical profession, as a whole, looked down on them as 'pen-pushers'. This was naturally resented by the civil servants, who, with some truth, thought of the senior medics as men of a narrow and self-interested vision who had got where they were frequently by parental influence. In addition, both Browne and Russell had been educated at English public schools, and on occasion displayed the arrogant self-assurance typical of that formation.

We have seen the results of some of the earlier skirmishes between the Department of Health and the Cancer Association. In 1954, just before the official opening of the hospital, James Deeny and another official, Owen Hargadon, were appointed to the Board of the Association, to replace T. J. Brady, Assistant Secretary of the Department who had in effect been hounded off the Board. (As a Departmental minute put it 'it became apparent that his presence as the Minister's representative at the Association's meetings was resented, and . . . his efforts were objectionable to certain members.'[28]) The Board was not happy with the new appointments, and indeed one might wonder if there was not an element of provocation. Deeny was not a career civil servant but a doctor, a Fellow of the Royal College of Physicians, with a strong vocational interest in public health. He was also the author of two detailed papers about cancer mortality in the Republic and so could reasonably claim some expertise in the matter.[29] He was a vigorous, outspoken man who was not easily intimidated. (He once chose a photograph of a very run-down school in the Archbishop of Dublin's own diocese as the cover image of a report on bad conditions in primary schools.) Chairman Ted Russell wrote a letter of protest about the appointments to James Ryan, to no effect.[30] For over a year the Board simply refused to recognise the new members' existence and the Secretary, Liam Egan, failed to inform them of meetings. This was probably illegal, and certainly a tactical error, since it gave the Department a ready stick with which to beat the Association.

In 1956 the Department, noting that St Luke's was, for its number of beds, one of the most expensive hospitals in Ireland, proposed that a British efficiency expert examine its operations. The Board, of course, refused, at least until the Minister laid down an ultimatum suggesting that if they did not concede he would cut off all funds. Now matters were coming to a head. It seemed to the Department that with three specialist hospitals and a large proportion of gastro-intestinal cancers being treated in general hospitals, there were more cancer beds than was required. With its large out-patient service, St Luke's in fact had only 67 per cent bed occupancy. One reason why there were more beds than was immediately needed was because the Consultative Cancer Council had based its estimate of the requirement on their proposal that St Anne's and Hume Street would in some way be folded into St Luke's. As we have seen, these hospitals continued to resist this idea, both actively and passively.

From 1957 Ted Russell and his colleague R. E. 'Bobby' Whelan began to take an increasingly uncompromising attitude, pushing the agenda of the Consultative Cancer Council report of 1949 to centralise state-wide cancer services on the Association. The Board representatives of both St Anne's and Hume Street (who had been appointed to the Board by Minister O'Higgins in an effort to speed up consolidation) began to express concern. As Deeny put it in an internal Departmental memo around this time, it was evident that a difficult situation in relation to cancer was brewing, one in which 'cooperation between the hospitals would be impossible.'

Over the next few months the atmosphere on the Board deteriorated. Whelan in particular seems to have become especially aggressive, his irritation apparently stimulated by the Department's practice, a function of its own cash problems, of putting off punctual payment of committed funds. This high-handed practice certainly made day-to-day running of the hospital very difficult.

The two Departmental representatives were subject to months of attack on the grounds of the Department's inefficiency, dishonesty and malpractice. At a meeting in April 1957 attended by the officials Whelan accused the Department of 'fraudulent practice and deliberate trickery' and complained 'that there was a conspiracy on the part of the Departmental officials to get the finances of the Association into a muddle'. Remonstrated with, Whelan declared that he was being as insulting as he knew how, presumably with a view to scaring the officials off the Board. [31] (Long after these events Russell described Whelan as 'a good friend of mine who, somewhat intemperate in his attitude to civil servants, did more than anyone to get things done'. [32])

In May 1957 the Secretary of the Department noted to the Minister that as long as Whelan stayed on the Board 'a serious and responsible approach to the problem [of the development of cancer services] will be quite impossible.' As result of this memo, in July R. E. Whelan left the Board. Ted Russell stayed for another two years.

In the summer of 1958 Deeny recorded that for the first time in over a hundred years there had been no new case of tuberculosis in Ireland for two successive months. The white plague was, it seemed, over. 'It took', as he recorded in his memoirs, 'a while to sink in.'

> Here was the tuberculosis epidemic, which had lasted for more than a hundred years and had killed more than three-quarters of a million Irish men, women and children and on which we had been working

for years, finally coming to an end. So far as I remember, we shook hands , but otherwise were in a kind of daze. There were no victory celebrations or parades; I don't think we even went out for a drink to mark the event.[33]

When he presented the results to a meeting of the Social and Statistical Society sometime later tuberculosis had become so much yesterday's story that a mere seven people turned up.

Driven in particular by Deeny, the Department had strongly focused on tuberculosis and it was no coincidence that very soon afterwards Deeny left the country to spend two years in Indonesia on behalf of the World Health Organisation. He resigned from the Board of the Cancer Association in September 1958.

In the meantime a serio-comic blunder had not improved relations. In May, Congressman John Fogarty, who was much involved in cancer and disability fundraising and administration in the United States,[34] was in Ireland. In the course of his visit he had met Seán MacEntee and reported the opinion in the United States that standards in Irish hospitals were low. Anxious to refute this, MacEntee had organised an immediate visit to St Luke's. Unfortunately, the arrangements were bungled.

Oliver Chance was on holiday, the Assistant Medical Director was attending a clinic in the west, and the only other senior doctor was looking after the out-patients' clinic. While the Secretary of the Department wandered around the hospital looking for help, the Minister and the Congressman sat in the car. Eventually they were shown into an office where they waited a further quarter of an hour before finally being escorted round the hospital. MacEntee, a notably vain man, felt himself humiliated in front of the Congressman.

He wrote an angry letter to Ted Russell (headed 'Dear Deputy', as Russell had become an Independent TD for Limerick in the March 1957 election) curtly pointing out how 'a reasonably well conducted establishment should have been able to arrange matters very much better.'[35] MacEntee declared that he had 'immediate responsibility for all hospital services' in Ireland and he was due more respect. The Chairman's response, though apologetic, spent much time recording successful visits from other experts. Not very tactfully he also remarked that 'in the final analysis it is our service to the patients that counts'.

It is perhaps not surprising that when, a few months later, Ted Russell proposed to meet the Minister for a 'man-to-man talk between us' about the affairs of the Association, he was rebuffed. Indeed, after a stiff exchange of letters, MacEntee decided to meet the members of the Association as a body and issued invitations to that effect. Russell and two other Board members declined to attend. At this meeting on 27 November MacEntee read out a long statement of his dissatisfaction with the current state of relations. His ultimate point, however, was that it was his responsibility under the Oireachtas to monitor the activities of the Association, and he was determined to do so.[36]

This face-off would perhaps be more entertaining than significant if the bad relations with the Department had not affected the Association's ability to achieve its goals. On one occasion, for instance, Ted Russell and a deputation visited the Department with a proposal that the Association engage in cancer research, and requested the Minister to provide funds to that end. Seán MacEntee not unreasonably asked for more detailed proposals. 'Alderman Russell', recorded a Departmental memo, 'informed the Minister that if he did not provide the money, the Association would be obliged to look elsewhere.'[37] This might include appeals for funds outside the country. Hackles up, the Minister refused both to provide any funds and to allow the Association to campaign outside Ireland (which might, in his view, negatively affect the Sweepstake income). The discussion degenerated into complaints from Russell about the 'pin-pricking' requests from the Department for financial information, and the possibility of funded cancer research was lost. As it happened, Russell was out of order in this. The Memorandum of the Cancer Association makes it clear that borrowing and raising money was one of the few potential activities that did require formal Ministerial consent.[38]

In the end the Department decided to dismantle for good the grand idea behind the Cancer Association. In a letter of May 1955 to Reggie Redmond, a personal friend who began his long association with the hospital by joining the Board at this time, MacEntee explained that, as the Department saw it, the Association had two main but distinct functions i.e. the administration of St Luke's Cancer Hospital and the 'furnishing of advice to the Minister on matters concerning the more general problem of the development and co-ordination of existing cancer services'.[39] The important further role envisaged by the Consultative Cancer Council's report, and taken seriously by Russell and his colleagues, which was the creation of a co-ordinated centre of excellence for the treatment of cancer across the state, was ignored.

MacEntee now proposed that the Cancer Association's functions be split into two. A new Board, which would not include representatives from Hume Street or St Anne's, would be solely concerned with running St Luke's. There was also to be established a permanent Consultative Council to provide advice to the Minister on cancer matters. Once again, no mention was made of the larger idea of a national centre for cancer.

The existing Board of the Cancer Association were asked to resign, and a completely new Board was appointed. The Department's view had prevailed, and its complete victory was signalled by the appointment of Owen Hargadon, one of the two officials who had been the centre of so much vituperation, as the new Chairman, a post he held until 1980. A mean little gesture accompanied the Department's victory. In the Association's *Report on the year 1959*, the new Board praises the contribution of the 'most active and valuable member' Mr H. M. Hughes, who had recently died. This is in deliberate and striking contrast to the bald way in which the report merely records that Russell and two others had 'resigned their membership of the Association'. The final act of the saga was the proposal that the Cancer Association, with its memories of large aspirations, be renamed simply St Luke's Hospital Ltd. This was effected in March 1961.

# Chapter 4: The Minister's hospital

St Luke's had been established partly so it could serve as the base for the investment required to maintain up-to-date radiation treatment of cancer. The hi-tech equipment involved was not only expensive to purchase, but also needed special staff to keep it in running order. Among these were newcomers to the hospital scene such as highly-qualified physicists. Unfortunately, the mindset of the Department of Health was unused to such large investments. So when St Luke's put forward its request for a high energy 'cobalt bomb' in 1958, a demand that had been envisaged by the report of the original Consultative Committee, it was to take several years and some prodding before a positive result was achieved.

When the hospital opened in 1954 the workings of the human cell were still very obscure (Crick and Watson's path-breaking paper on the structure of DNA was only published in April 1953.) However, radiologists knew that, as one practitioner's publication put it, 'exposure to penetrating radiation from specially designed sources is one of the simplest ways of altering the growth conditions of living cells'.[1] In other words, it was a good way first to prevent tumours growing and then to kill the cells that made them up. Exactly how this was thought to happen was still unclear. It was explained that radiation first 'holds up temporarily a proportion of dividing cells from entering mitosis'. A few hours later, when mitotic activity [cell division] resumes, so-called degenerate cells 'break down on attempting division'. Thus radiation could prevent malignant cells from dividing, and it would ultimately eradicate the tumour. Very high doses of radiation, outside the normal therapeutic range, had the effect of simply killing all cells within range. It was understood that the relatively simple malignant cells were more susceptible to this effect than more differentiated ones. A problem arose because radiation treatment also unavoidably damaged the blood vessels surrounding the tumour, and this indirect effect in itself could lead to 'massive destruction among the cells of the tissue involved'. The idea of removing the supply of blood from a tumour was to re-emerge as a way of attacking cancer in the 1980s.

Clearly, x-rays damaged healthy and malignant cells almost equally. So the radiologist's problem was to deliver these effects to the affected area with the least possible damage to surrounding normal tissues. The mainstays of current radiotherapy were, first, the so-called 'superficial' x-ray machines in the 60-120kV range providing a dose adequate for skin cancers and those no more than one or two centimetres below the skin. The workhorses of St Luke's radiotherapy were four 'deep' x-ray machines, using 200–250kV, used to attack more sunken tumours. Unfortunately, they were not capable of penetrating more than about 10 centimetres (4 inches) below the surface without excessive irradiation of surrounding tissues.[2]

The next stage was to acquire a high energy device which would penetrate to tumours sunk more deeply into the body; in addition, dosing with high energy devices was often more accurate, and less uncomfortable for the patients. Patients were already being sent to England for this kind of treatment. Obviously, St Luke's needed some such device—the question was which would be best? The choice was between one of the new super-voltage linear accelerator x-ray machines or a machine using radio-active cobalt—the so-called 'cobalt bomb'. John O'Connor, the hospital's Chief Physicist, was clear that the linear accelerator was in some ways the better machine: it could deliver large amounts of radiation in a short time, thus enabling the unit to handle more patients in a day. Also it would not require to be regularly supplied with expensive radioactive material. The decisive point against the linear accelerator, however, was the cost. The basic unit was twice as dear as the rival cobalt bomb and required a full-time maintenance engineer in attendance, not to mention the special housing required because of the use of high tension electricity. (The long process and eventual acquisition of a linear accelerator was a saga of the 1970s.)

The decision being made in favour of cobalt, the architect was asked to draw up plans for the housing of the new unit. He provided a provisional estimate in November 1957, so that John O'Connor was able to report to the Medical Director that the whole unit would cost some £20,000 (equivalent to €650,000 in today's currency). In April 1958 the Minister gave agreement in principle, subject to agreements being thrashed out with St Anne's and Hume Street for their use of the facility where reasonable. After considerable discussion (knotty questions arising such as who would be responsible for patients visiting St Luke's from the other hospitals, how and with what priority would they be booked in, and, of course, what would happen to the fees from private patients), agreement was apparently reached and in November 1959 Seán MacEntee announced in the Dáil that 'it is anticipated that the unit will be in operation before the end of the coming year'.[3]

For reasons which are not entirely clear, activity thereafter slowed to a snail's pace. No doubt St Luke's requirements were particular, and required some unusual features; no doubt the Department felt itself required to check every change on every detailed plan (on one occasion helpfully pointing out that 'no lighting or ventilation to the WC has been shown'[4]); perhaps this was necessary as the costs crept upwards—by 1961 tenders ranged from £32,000 to £36,000. However, things were only creeping forward, and faced daily with patients who could benefit from these machines, senior people in St Luke's began to get impatient. Why, they wanted to know, was it taking so long to install the cobalt machine?

*Oliver Chance retires*

In January 1961 the *Sunday Review* splashed a story claiming that 'somebody has been preventing Irish cancer patients from getting vital treatment.' 'We asked the Department of Health the reason for the delay', the article continued, 'we did so because 5,000 a year die from cancer and thousands must undergo severe treatment AND because one member of the Cancer Association of Ireland told us bluntly: "Government red tape is responsible".'[5] The Minister was of course very annoyed by this story, and immediately attacked the

Association. They in turn vigorously denied that 'any member of the Association' had made any such statement.

This response was more clever than wise. There were only six people who could be technically described as members of the Association, that is, the members of the Board. For different reasons none of them was at all likely to present such a story to the Sunday newspapers. Everyone, including the Department, knew or suspected that it was the Medical Director, Oliver Chance (technically an employee), who had made the statement. On 19 February the *Sunday Review* confirmed that their 'very reliable' informant was indeed not a member of the Association. However, perhaps things were speeded up as a result, for the contract was finally signed and sealed on 15 February. Even then the project seemed somewhat delay-prone, since in May a strike hit the cement factory in Drogheda; however, by special concession the union agreed to allow enough cement to leave the factory for this 'matter of national concern' as Liam Egan put it.

A year later the cobalt unit was still not treating patients. In the Dáil MacEntee was asked again when the unit would be in operation. 'The detailed arrangements,' he said evasively, 'are primarily matters for the authorities of the hospital. I am informed, however, that they expect to have the unit brought into operation for the treatment of patients in about three months' time.'[6] In fact the machine was in place in the hospital, but was being 'tuned' by the physicist John O'Connor. Soon after that patients were receiving the benefits.

But not patients from Hume Street or St Anne's, who both maintained their 'arm's length' attitude to St Luke's. Three attempts had been made to set up a liaison meeting, but, as the Board was told in July 1963, no one from those hospitals had attended. In December 1963 the Board was informed that neither hospital had sent any patients at all to take advantage of the new facilities in St Luke's. Of course, it is entirely possible that no appropriate patients had been available. However, a cynic might be tempted to wonder if the institutional resistance of these hospitals had in practice removed that option from the range of the possible, regardless of the patients' need. (Years later some consultants of St Luke's showed a similar reluctance to use unique equipment based, to their annoyance, in St Anne's.) The Board of St Luke's, on the other hand, was so happy with the unit that they were actively considering establishing one in St Agatha's in Cork, and in 1964 ordered a second machine for Dublin.

By this time relations between the Board and the Medical Director had deteriorated. Although Chance was not formally a member, as a matter of practice he participated in all Board meetings and received full minutes. However, his action in leaking the cobalt bomb story had no doubt made their relations with the Department difficult, and in 1963 he again seriously annoyed his fellow directors. This arose during a dispute about the appointment of a surgical consultant to the hospital.

The story illustrates an unhappy side to the small pond that was Dublin of the early 1960s. In the course of a bad-tempered dispute between MacEntee and the Irish Medical Association (which was nothing to do with the hospital), the Editor of the IMA's *Journal* wrote about the Minister's 'formidable escort' at some function, a comment which was interpreted as a rude reference to the Minister's wife, a lady the historian Ruth Barrington has described as of 'generous proportions'. MacEntee was not unreasonably furious. Since it was well known that Bob O'Connell, the surgeon favoured by Chance, was closely associated with the IMA, there was no possibility that he would be appointed. Although the appointment of personnel was in fact one of the few Board functions that were not 'subject to the consent of the Minister', the Board as it was then constituted was very unlikely to go against his preferences. On the other hand Chance, who was after all the Medical Director, insisted that his preferred candidate should be appointed, regardless of the political background.

A sub-committee was established to examine the numerous applications and Chance and a medical colleague out-voted Reggie Redmond, the lay member representing the Board. When it next met, the Board (two out of five of the other members of which were employees of the Department) over-ruled the sub-committee and offered the job elsewhere.

In an ill-considered attempt to nullify the Board's decision (for how could he possibly win in the long run?) at the next meeting Chance quoted clause 9(d) of the Articles to the effect that a member would cease to be a member of the Board 'if he absents himself from six consecutive meetings'. He pointed out that Mrs Jenny Dowdall, one-time Lord Mayor of Cork, had been absent, from a combination of sickness and political involvement, at least that time. Since she had consequently forfeited her right to vote, the whole decision, he argued, was null. This aggressive action was not taken well. In April 1963 the Board resolved that 'the Secretary is to write to the Medical Director expressing grave disapproval of an attempt by him to question the validity of a decision of the Board of Directors'. At the same meeting it was decided that he would no longer be sent the minutes of Board meetings and would only be invited to attend those parts specifically to do with medical matters.

Not long afterwards, in February 1968, Dr Chance reached his 65th birthday and a few months later retired. When he died in August 1972 (a few weeks before the ill-fated Munich Olympics) his obituarist noted that after his retirement from St Luke's he continued to hold clinics in St Anne's, his old stamping ground, and became active on the advisory committee of the Irish Cancer Society. 'We are entering', he was quoted as saying, 'the era of positive health, and people should think more of preventing disease and eliminating the circumstances which made its occurrence possible.' Somewhat unrealistically, considering how many potential cancers there are, he proposed that everyone over thirty or forty should have regular examinations every three or five years for signs of cancer.[7]

### The new St Luke's

The row about the appointment of a surgeon consultant reflects a sea-change in the attitude of the Board. In 1961 the Memorandum and Articles had been revised. Most obviously the name had been changed from the Cancer Association to St Luke's. Less apparent was the series of amendments that added the restriction 'subject to the consent of the Minister' to almost any potential action. The Department was not going to be run away with again. The six-person Board now consisted of Owen Hargadon and Malachy Powell from the Department, Reggie Redmond, Senator Mrs Jenny Dowdall, Professor Kearney from Cork and Dr Neans de Paor. This new Board saw St Luke's as very much 'the Minister's hospital'— even to the extent of refusing to cooperate with the Irish Cancer Society when it was founded in 1963, on the grounds that St Luke's ought to remain above the fray.

There was no obvious successor to Oliver Chance. A radiotherapist was clearly required, and there was no apparent possibility outside St Luke's unless they went abroad, a much more radical procedure then than now. The problem was that, of the three consultants based in Dublin, Michael O'Halloran was considered too young; Finbarr Cross was not a well man (and indeed was later to spend some months recuperating in a private ward of the hospital); and John Healy was regarded as something of a maverick. Stories were told of how he ignored the taxis laid on to take him to the country clinics and insisted on flying his private plane. He was regularly scolded by the Board for impulsive actions. On one occasion he used St Luke's headed notepaper to send a circular to doctors in Dublin about a trial he was conducting; on another he organised a lecture in Galway in association with the Irish Cancer Society without the Board's permission. And then there was a mysterious 'incident' in which he was involved; this nearly led to his suspension, but Liam Egan's discreet minutes give no further details. (He was also, though the Board did not consider this, perhaps the patients' best-loved doctor of his generation.)

Puzzled as to who to select as Chance's replacement, the Board established a triumvirate. The idea was that each of the Dublin consultants would be acting medical director for a year in rotation. Elaborate arrangements were set out for a committee of the four consultant radiotherapists, to be chaired in rotation. Seán MacEntee warned that this would not work, and it did not. Eventually, in 1973 the board appointed Michael O'Halloran as Medical Director, a post he held until 1988.

# A Haven in Rathgar—St Luke's

## *Thinking about cancer*

One of the hardest things in medical history is to understand how people in the past, even a generation ago, thought about and suffered disease, pain and death. Because what people think so much affects what they feel, we cannot be sure either exactly how the tastes of food, the consolations of religion or the tenderness of sex were experienced. Words become slippery, and change power and meaning over a generation, and even depending on who is in the conversation. Not wanting to 'make a fuss', this person mentions only 'feeling tired', and being 'uncomfortable'; another, frightened, wanting reassurance, is 'exhausted, sleepless' and 'in quite a lot of pain'. Objectively, one can imagine that deep bone pain in cancer is at one extreme of pain, with normal back-ache at the other. But one person can never know what another feels especially when fear is in the soul. In this context it is interesting that for many of its patients St Luke's, at least in the early days, saw pain as the enemy. 'Most of the tumours with which we dealt', wrote Oliver Chance, 'were such that the likelihood of cure was remote; in fact all one expected was palliation'.[8]

It is usually impossible to recreate the intimate world of the patient and doctor. However, cancer is, in this as in other things, special. It is evident that the diagnosis of cancer provides people with a kind of existential blow that they very often feel the need to communicate. As an Irish author put it : 'Cancer alters your whole outlook; you feel as though you have moved to another plane, a place where only those with this possible death sentence live and understand you. I wrote my story, I suppose, so people could get inside my head and see what it is really like to go through cancer.'[9]

In recent years in particular, cancer has become unique among diseases in having so large a literature written by patients. Tuberculosis has been more glamourised by professional writers. When novelists mention cancer at all it has tended to be obliquely, and a matter of secrets, as when, in *The Grapes of Wrath* Sairy Wilson refuses to tell her husband what her sickness means: 'I'm jus' pain covered with skin. I know what it is, but I won't tell him. He'd be too sad. He wouldn't know what to do anyways.'[10]

In 1978 the American critic Susan Sontag attacked this glamourisation and also modern attitudes to cancer as blunting our responses to these diseases by hiding them behind metaphors of sickness.[11] This influential essay has perhaps been instrumental in encouraging the proliferation of autobiographical accounts of cancer which have appeared since. It appears that the experience of cancer has pushed many ordinary people into writing, often very movingly, of their brush with the disease. Much of this literature is apparently written to encourage fellow-sufferers, and to work through the stigma of being host to such a disease. Ferdia MacAnna, writing in the mid-1980s about his encounter with testicular cancer, wrote:

> One of the best things about being in Vincent's was that I could talk about cancer without feeling guilty or paranoid. In hospital I didn't feel like a freak. Outside it was almost impossible to discuss my problem. At the mention of the word cancer people grew uneasy and either changed the subject or found an excuse to leave. It got to the point where I began to feel ashamed of having cancer. My cancer was dirty, uncivilised, bad manners, impolite, disgusting, contagious, fatal, . . . unpleasant. It reminded people of their own frail mortality.[12]

In Ireland this literature starts in the 1960s, with John McGahern's *The Barracks*, a moving novel about a police sergeant's wife with breast cancer. McGahern records how Elizabeth Reegan 'knew she must see a doctor, but she had known that months before, and she'd done nothing. She'd first discovered the cysts last August . . . and she remembered her fright and incomprehension when she touched her right breast again with the towel.'[13] A report in *The Irish Times* in January 1955 confirmed that this reluctance to hear the bad news was common. A study in Manchester showed that half of women questioned assumed cancer was incurable, and three-quarters had never heard of the case of a cure. Because they assumed it was hopeless, many women tended to delay seeking medical attention, thus significantly worsening their prognosis.

At any one time cancer patients and those not affected hold a wide variety of ideas about cancer. There are those up to date with the latest fashionable scientific and medical opinions (which, of course, vary themselves from decade to decade—now cancer is caused by pollutants, now viruses, now hereditable mutations, and so on). At the other end of this spectrum, there is a strange fauna of half-understood ideas, often regurgitations of obsolete medical opinions. In between these extremes are people who, while professing broadly correct medical ideas, retain an obstinate affection for this superstition or that bit of folklore. Ideas about cancer are typically not 'joined up' into a coherent theory. Traditional opinions, the favourite theories of the local GP, half-remembered articles in magazines, class and religious prejudices all stir into the mix.

In the 1960s Mary Feehan, Cork-based publisher Seán Feehan's 38-year-old wife, had had two successive operations for benign lumps, and then, fatally, just stopped going for regular checks. The next lump discovered was also under her arm, and was both malignant and spreading. After an operation in a Cork nursing home, the specialist summoned her husband to his office, in the style of the day telling the next-of-kin before the patient: 'The news is not good. As yet it is hard to say how far it has gone, but just to be on the safe side I propose to operate again in a few days and remove her ovaries . . . then I propose to put her on radiation treatment after the operation, and we will see how that works.' To his shock and horror, Seán Feehan realised that his beloved wife probably had no more than five years to live, and he was suddenly faced with the intractable losing lottery of the disease.

The available weapons to combat cancer were not many. In 1954 *The Bell* spoke of three treatments, surgery, which is 'often completely successful', treatment with gamma-rays or x-rays which 'often has decisive results', and finally, the author notes, 'encouraging, if not definitive results have recently been obtained through chemical treatment.' Noting that cancer is 'one of the very few maladies which does not heal itself', the author sternly rejects all other treatments. This includes magnetic passes, incantations, nature cures and homeopathy. Indeed 'such charlatanism is fatal because it delays recourse to a qualified specialist and can transform a cancer, curable at the beginning, into an inevitably fatal illness.'[14]

A sample from the magazine *Woman's Way*, from the 'Patient's Postbag' of 1970, makes it clear that quite vague ideas and fears about carcinogenesis prevailed. One asks 'Are painful periods a sign of cancer of the womb?' Another echoes a common fear: 'My problem is how to disinfect a room where my brother was nursed for many months. He died of cancer of the stomach. I have a family and feel it may be dangerous to use the room without having it thoroughly disinfected.' The doctor answered: 'Cancer is not infectious in the way you describe. Have the room painted and freshly papered.' Another asks about rectal bleeding: 'is it likely to turn into cancer?' (*Ans*: 'No, it is almost certainly just piles'); another wants to know about the exercises she is doing to enlarge her breasts: 'Will I damage my bust with these exercises? I am afraid of cancer.' (*Ans.* 'Don't worry, that is not how cancer works').

As time went on people allowed themselves to talk more publicly of cancer.[15] An important influence was Rachel Carson's pioneering environmental awareness book *Silent Spring*, which was published in 1962. In the chapter ominously called 'One in every four' she pictured the threat to American families embodied in increasing use of pesticides, herbicides and other man-made chemicals. Sensationally, she declared that these chemicals would cause a massive upsurge of cancers, which she predicted would affect as many as 45 million victims. (The US population was no more than 200 million at the time.)

Throughout the 1960s a growing campaign, driven by the widow of advertising mastermind Albert Lasker, promoted 'the fight against cancer'. 'If the American people can accept the placing of a man on the moon and similar projects as important national goals', they argued, 'surely finding a cure or control for cancer is a reasonable and worthwhile national goal.' Over-persuaded by scientists, the campaign constantly stressed that 'we are on the verge of' some great progress—sometimes it was a cure, sometimes only 'important advances.' Newspapers and magazines regularly announced 'Cancer breakthrough', or 'Cancer: has the tide turned?' To which, of course, the answer was No—but that was not what their readers wanted to hear. The rhetoric was often irresponsible: 'Cancer is one of the most curable of the major diseases in this country' declared one pamphlet issued by the American Cancer Society in 1971. In 1969 Mrs Lasker and her team took out a full page ad in the New York Times declaring MR. NIXON, YOU CAN CURE CANCER. He took the bait. In 1971 he promoted through Congress the so-called 'War against Cancer' hoping perhaps to draw to himself some of the prestige that Roosevelt's successful March of the Dimes against polio had garnered. Unfortunately for Nixon, slick rhetoric about space exploration was easily turned against him. As one critic pointed out, landing a man on the moon would have been impossible before scientists had understood Newton's law of gravitation, and that was the equivalent state of knowledge about the mechanics of cancer inside the cell. Nonetheless it was difficult for Congress to be against cancer research, and enormous sums of money were allocated.

Critics quickly pointed out that this cornucopia of money had merely created a medical research gravy train and a bureaucracy which supported the established researchers and effectively stifled creativity. The war analogy turned sour too, as reporters likened the effort more to Vietnam than an American triumph. One commentator opined cynically: 'More people were making a living off cancer than ever died of it.' This was a gross exaggeration, but there is no doubt that the huge bulk of research funds went to projects following established lines in virology, immunology, chemotherapy and radiation; out of $581 million spent in 1974, a mere $2.7 million went on preventive nutrition research.

The campaign was undoubtedly further stimulated by well-publicised studies associating the growing mortality from cancer with a list of everyday industrial chemicals. Chief among these was cigarette smoke, but the frightening thing was that even if one did not smoke and avoided passively inhaling, there was, as one researcher declared, an enormous and unavoidable range of plastics, dyes, solvents, resins, lacquers, paints, building materials, textile fibres, motor fuels and food components that were potentially carcinogenic.[16]

More or less everything, it seemed, could cause cancer. In 1977 a science writer in the *New York Times* wrote: 'The average person in modern societies lives in a veritable sea of carcinogens. The air we breathe, the food we eat, the drugs we take, the water we drink, the clothing we wear, all may contain substances that have been shown to cause cancer in animals or man.' Furthermore, the Environment Protection Agency declared that 'there is no such thing as a safe level of exposure' to any carcinogen—thus completely ignoring, for instance, fifty years' experience of skilled radiologists. To add to the mood, CBS announced (wrongly) that America was the most cancer-prone society in the world. Not surprisingly perhaps, as one leading medical writer pointed out, 'when it comes to cancer, American society is far from rational. We are possessed by fear . . . cancer-phobia has expanded into a demonism in which the evil spirit is ever present, but furtively viewed and spoken of obliquely.'

This feeling was no doubt behind President Lyndon Johnson's denial of his successful treatment for skin cancer on his ankle in 1967, a denial persevered in by his family years after his death.

At the same time, in the 1970s the theory of the 'cancer personality' emerged. Stemming from research into heart disease, this quickly led to an exaggerated sense that patients were in control of their physical destiny. The ancient Greeks used to say 'none could be called happy until that day when he carries his happiness down to the grave in peace'.[17] To the moderns it seemed as if *anything* was preferable to being dead. This sentiment drove doctors to so-called 'heroic' treatments, and for 'can-do' Americans it seemed in some obscure way *their fault* if the disease was allowed the upper hand.

The importance of morale in medical care is an old line of thinking, traceable in the old Roman physician Galen, but was given a new lease of life by the US psychologist L. LeShan who in a series of studies in the 1950s and 1960s found that a high proportion of cancer patients suffered from a basic inability to express emotion, which led to 'growing despair'. This was 'strongly connected with the loss [of affectionate relationships] that each had suffered in childhood'. These unfortunates died, so it was said, much more readily than their psychologically robust fellow patients.[18] LeShan, in a popular book, declared appealingly *You can fight for your life.*

The attraction of this junk science combined a sense that patients were in charge of their lives (difficult to achieve when seriously zapped by drugs or radiation), with suspicions of 'big medicine'. In hospitals a positive attitude was encouraged: 'Nurse Mary reminded me,' writes Ferdia MacAnna of his time in St Vincent's, 'that will-power was important. "I've seen people beat cancers that were a lot worse than yours. They just kept on fighting" she told me.'[19] The fact that no one in the so-called 'cancer establishment' had a good theory of tumoro-genesis merely proved, it was argued, how far they had gone down the wrong track. Despite eloquent refutation from orthodox practitioners and writers such as Susan Sontag, the door opened to a rich flora of well-meaning or exploitative quacks. The descendants of those who in the 1900s had declared that with ancient recipes derived from native tribes 'we can cure tuberculosis' now declared that, using ancient meditation techniques, 'we can cure cancer'.

One thing everyone agreed upon was that if the patient delayed or if the cancer had advanced too far, there was little that could be done. In the memoir *I'm not afraid to die,* published in 1974, the author, identified merely as 'An Irish housewife' tells of how 'a lump had appeared on my back, for no apparent reason. Naturally I headed to [her GP]. That visit was followed by tests, injections, x-rays and more tests, more injections and more tests. Then pain became my constant companion.' Eventually the last set of x-rays comes back from examination by a specialist in Dublin: '"Ellen," the GP began, "the news is not so good this time . . . of course they are trying out new drugs all the time, but an operation would be out of the question even now."' Interestingly there had been no mention of drugs in Mary Feehan's case, or in Elizabeth Reegan's in *The Barracks,* reflecting the fact that this memoir was published a few years after the others. Unfortunately, there was apparently no question of radiation treatment: the housewife is told she had 'eighteen months to two years at the outside' to live.

Eventually self-diagnosis reaches its limits. Elizabeth Reegan is forced by pain and growing tiredness to visit her GP. McGahern touches on the multiple responses elicited by our self-conscious bodies that can make the medical encounter so problematic, even agonisingly embarrassing, for the patient: 'The breasts that men had desired to touch by instinct and to seek their own sensual dreams of her there, now these professional hands sought their objective knowledge of her, for a living.' A correspondent to *Woman's Way* in 1970 wrote of how she was embarrassed to speak to the doctor of her rectal bleeding. She was hopefully reassured by the doctor 'this is usually associated with piles. There is no need to feel embarrassed, as doctors deal with such things every day.'[20] This embarrassment was not of course exclusively or perhaps, if truth were known, mainly female. Ferdia MacAnna records how 'some people wanted to know what kind of cancer I had, but I was afraid to tell them the truth. "Testicular cancer" sounded so shameful, as though I was about to lose my private parts altogether through some fault of my own . . . I told people I had abdominal cancer. It was a more serious form of cancer, but somehow it sounded less immediately threatening to my manhood.'[21]

Elisabeth Reegan's doctor spoke. '"I don't think you have a thing to worry about, but," and she knew the words that were coming. "from my examination it'd be better to send you for a hospital investigation, just to make certain."' She spends some days in the County Hospital, undergoing tests, and then 'they had taken the biopsy of the breast and sent it to Dublin for analysis. The final diagnosis had come back: she had cancer.'

In the local hospital the specialist, from a good school, with his 'man's hand-tailored suit and greying hair, the formal kindness of his voice' tells the husband that 'she'd have to go to Dublin to have an operation . . . if the operation proved successful she might live for ten or more years.' If not, a year or perhaps two was all that might be expected. The husband, a garda sergeant who had been active in the civil war, feels about the encounter, with its strong overtones of class difference, as if his wife has been taken over by a remorseless scientific experiment.

A few days later she arrives in St Luke's, a hospital as McGahern put it, in the suburbs of Dublin, with the tree-bordered avenue, the lodge gate with two round lamps on the piers, and a fine view of the mountains. St Luke's, 'new state hospital, modern and American, several rectangles of flat roofs in geometric design, the walls more glass than concrete', is described sympathetically.

The impression gained by nine-year-old Robin Heron, diagnosed at that time with lympho-sarcoma, was equally favourable. His relationship with St Luke's, disguised in Inez Heron's account of the events as 'Bramble Grange',[22] started well. 'Dr Monaghan', described as 'with a thin vulpine face and a gentle unassuming manner' arranged to have the child transferred. '"Would you be willing to come to my hospital, Robin?" he asked "We specialise in curing pain."' After his experiences with repeated surgery and sadly inadequate pain control in 'Holy Innocents' Hospital, this was welcome. On arrival Robin was put into a private room 'on the top floor of a two-storey wing. "No 12 Wing P" midway down a corridor which opened from the nurses' station . . . outside, patients in dressing-gowns were enjoying the sunshine. A small child sat in a wheelchair, shaded by an almond tree.'

Inez Heron, Robin's mother, quickly found her way around St Luke's, and has left us a description of how it felt at the time.

> It was a small hospital: one hundred and fifty beds. The turnover was fairly quick. In the old mansion there was a hostel for ambulatory patients domiciled outside the city. Once their treatment was completed for the day they were free to go out to visit friends, go shopping in town or wander down to the local pubs.
>
> It was generously staffed. Ward P carried a ratio of 15 nurses to 20 patients. Allowing for off-duty and holiday periods it meant that only rarely were they working under pressure. Ward orderlies helped with bed making, serving meals and routine patient care . . .
>
> The emphasis was on the patients' mental and physical welfare. The relief of pain was the first priority, to rehabilitate patients for a return to as full and normal a life as possible.'

The next day Robin has his first session of deep x-ray treatment (DXT).

> Robin was pushed along to the Radiotherapy Department. A bright airy hall with small changing cubicles and several x-ray treatment rooms . . . Robin was 'screened'. Details were filled in on a treatment sheet; notations of the area to be treated and the dose of cobalt to be

administered, The skin was marked with blue outlines.

An attractive radiotherapist, in a trim-fitting white coat, then took Robin to the treatment room. He was lifted on to the table and settled comfortably. It was a sealed room, artificially lighted, with a glass window through which she could watch him.

The overhead x-ray machine was adjusted. Her friendly chat dispelled any apprehension Robin might have had. She placed a push-bell near his hand in case he wanted to call her during treatment.

I followed her out. Robin looked round with interest. The door was closed. She settled herself on a swivel chair at the controls of her plant. She clicked various switches, lights illuminated the dials. Through the window panel I could see Robin lying quite still. In less than a minute it was over. Wrapped in his dressing gown he was lifted back into the wheelchair.

Dr Monaghan spoke cheerfully. 'That wasn't too bad, now was it, Robin?'

But lest her readers should be deceived by this mildness, Inez Heron adds: 'Always after every treatment, he vomited. Like seasickness, it was preceded by nausea. Then a single bout of vomiting.'

After several courses of radium the confident diagnosis of the surgeon at 'Holy Innocents'—'massive growth on the back abdominal wall'—began to be doubted. The fact that the supposed cancer was not spreading in the expected way made the staff in 'Bramble Grange' suspicious. 'If it had been lymphosarcoma', one told Robin's mother, 'there would have been metastatis—migration to other areas. Multiple growths. It is almost impossible that Robin could have survived these last months without further eruptions.' After further tests, involving, of course, more discomfort and pain for young Robin, the final diagnosis was not cancer at all, but the parasitic disease Toxicariasis, which was then regarded as uncommon if not rare. Ultimately, after much further trauma, this was cured by drugs.

'You know,' said Inez Heron to one of the doctors, reflecting on Robin's very difference experience there and in 'Holy Innocents'.

Bramble Grange is so different to the average hospitals. The fear structure doesn't exist here. The sort of situation where consultants are revered as oracles, I mean. Where the housemen are overworked and always in a hurry dealing with crises; and the nurses-in-training are in terror of the staff sisters. Here it's a cooperative effort; and there's this extraordinary honesty, even about your divergence of views.

At the end of her emotional book about her son's devastating sickness and ultimate recovery, Inez Heron wrote a moving tribute to the medical staff of St Luke's:

> Robin was lucky—and we were lucky too—that at Bramble Grange we found a team who would not accept defeat. We owe them a debt which can never be repaid, for they gave the gift of life. They won because they refused to lose.

That was a good day for St Luke's.

# St Luke's in pictures

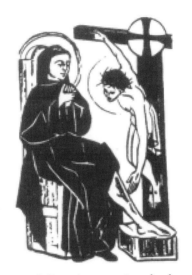

*St Peregrine was miraculously
cured of a tumour on his
leg in 1325. He was
named patron saint
of cancer sufferers
in 1726.*

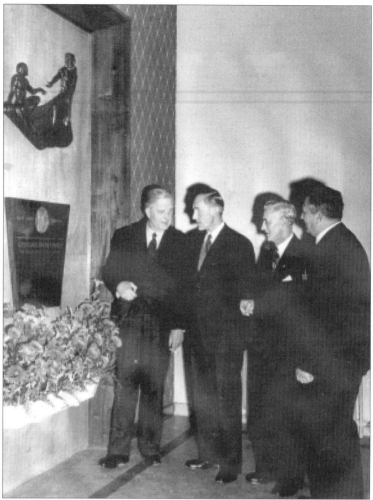

*The first opening, in October 1952—(left to right) James Ryan, Minister for Health, Ted Russell, Cancer Association Chairman, Andy Clarkin, Lord Mayor of Dublin, and Dr Oliver Chance, Medical Director*

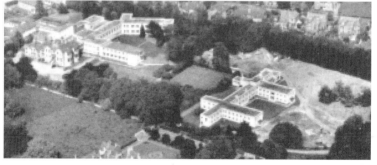

*Aerial view from the 1950s shows (right) the original nurses' home, now Oakland Lodge, and (left) the new hospital stretching behind the old house. The original entrance to the hospital was between the old house and the new building.*

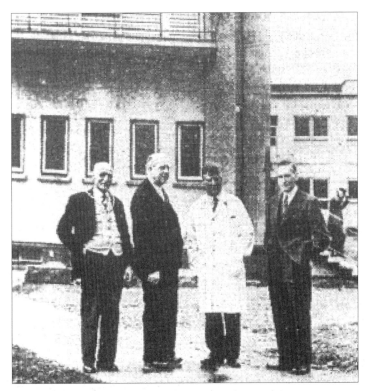

*The formal opening in May 1954, with the hospital still something of a building site—(left to right) James Butler, Lord Mayor of Dublin, James Ryan, Minister for Health, Dr Oliver Chance, Medical Director, Ted Russell, Chairman Cancer Association*

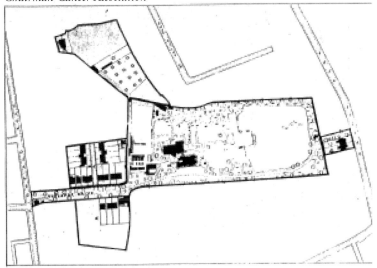

*The original estate agent's map showing the extent of the land purchase between Highfield Road and Orwell Park*

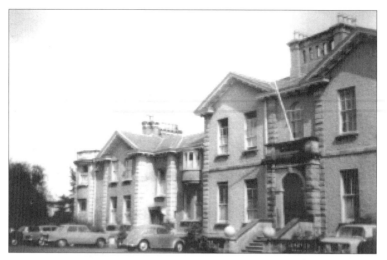

*The house as it was when the Cancer Association bought it. The original house is on the right, with the stairs flanked by two windows on either side. The cars on the left are parked in front of the extension added by the Hely family.*

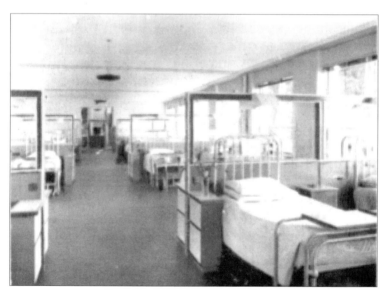

*The original ward design broke the wards into groups of eight beds, but visibility was more marked than privacy.*

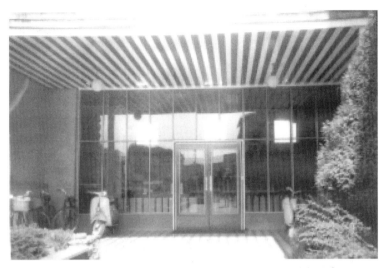

*The original entrance to the hospital, now the side entrance to Ward D.*

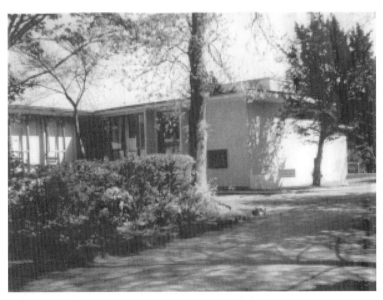

*The out-patients' entrance in 1953—architect Thomas Kennedy won the Gold Medal of the Royal Institute of Architects of Ireland for the design.*

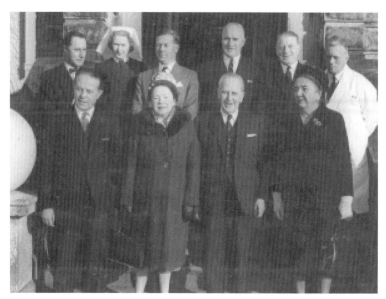

*The Minister's visit 18 November 1959—*
*front (left to right) Owen Hargadon,Chairman, Dr Neans de Paor, Seán*
*MacEntee, Minister for Health, Senator Mrs Jenny Dowdall*
*back (left to right) Liam Egan, Secretary-Registrar, Mary Dixon, Matron,*
*Reggie Redmond, Paddy Murray, Secretary of the Department of Health, Dr*
*Malachy Powell, Dr Oliver Chance, Medical Director*

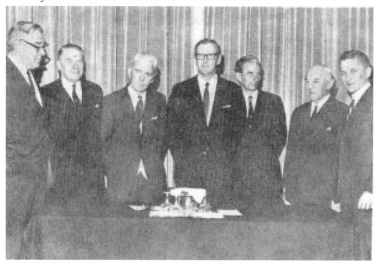

*At a seminar on cancer in Cork 1967—*
*(left to right) Dr F. H. Cross, Dr Malachy Powell, Dr M. Bennett, Dr*
*Michael O'Halloran, Dr John O'Connor, Prof. R. A. Q. O'Meara, Dr John*
*Healy*

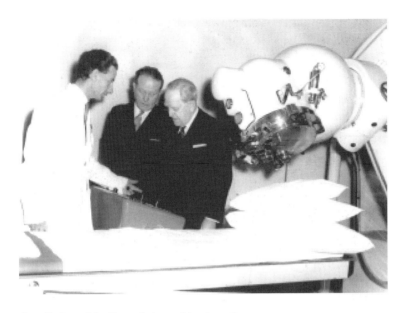

*Installation of the first cobalt machine in 1962—*
*(left to right) Dr John O'Connor, Chief Physicist, Owen Hargadon, Chair-*
*man and Seán MacEntee, Minister for Health*

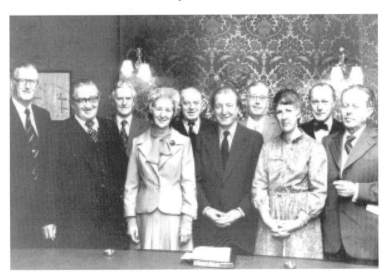

*Celebrating the hospital's 25th anniversary, 23 November 1979—*
*(left to right) Dr Michael O'Halloran, Dr Bryan Alton, Brendan Hensey*
*(Secretary of the Department of Health) Esther Byrne, Secretary-Manager,*
*Dr Malachy Powell, Charles Haughey, Reggie Redmond, Margaret Johnston,*
*Matron, Liam Egan, Owen Hargadon, Chairman*

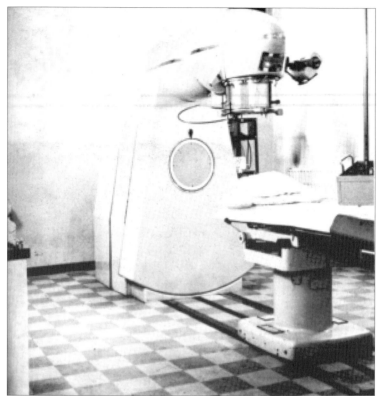

*The hospital's second cobalt machine was installed in St Agatha's Clinic in Cork which later became part of Cork University Hospital.*

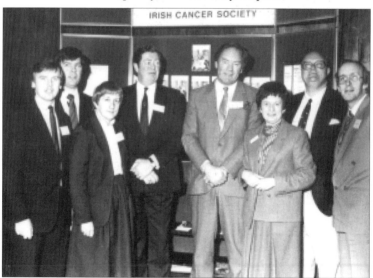

*At a meeting of the Irish Cancer Society in 1987—(left to right) Dr Peter Daly, Dr Des Carney, Sr Margaret McMenamin, Charlie Culley (the initator of Daffodil Day), Dr James Fennelly, Avril Gilliat, Dr Tim McElwaine from UK, Dr Michael Moriarty (courtesy Dr Peter Daly)*

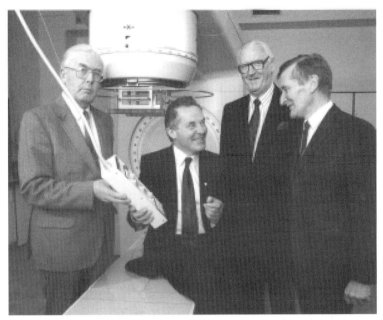

*Celebrating the installation of the third Linac in November 1989—
(left to right) Reggie Redmond, Chairman, Dr Rory O'Hanlon, Minister for
Health, Dr Michael O'Halloran, Dr John Healy*

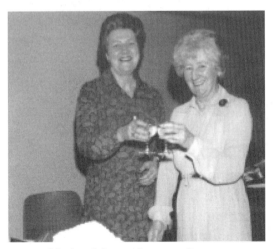

*Kay Rochford with her predecessor as Secretary-
Manager Esther Byrne on the latter's retirement in 1983*

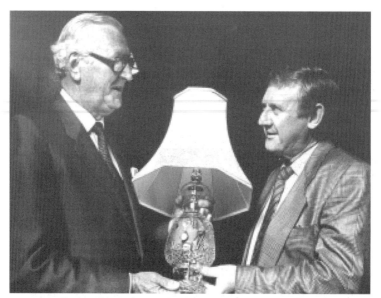

*Dr Michael O'Halloran, initiator and first Chairman of the Friends of St Luke's, and Niall Tobin at a fundraiser in the 1980s*

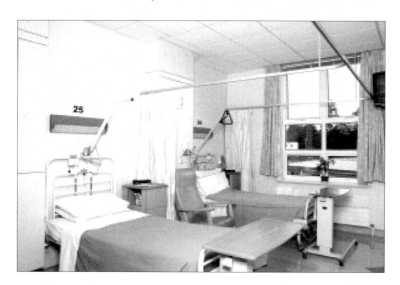

*A modern ward*

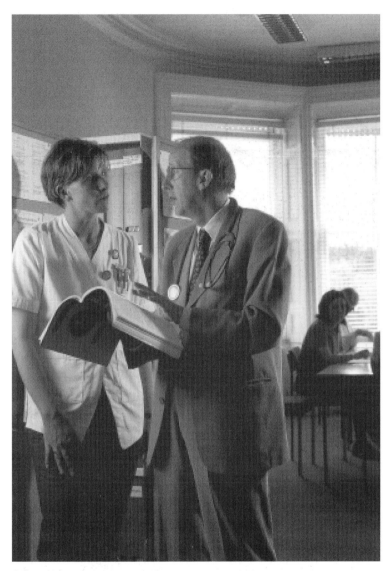

*Dr Michael Moriarty, seen here in the Resource Centre with Nurse Nuala Cody, was Chief of Radiotherapy and Oncology 1992–5. He was a critical influence in sustaining the ethos of the hospital.*

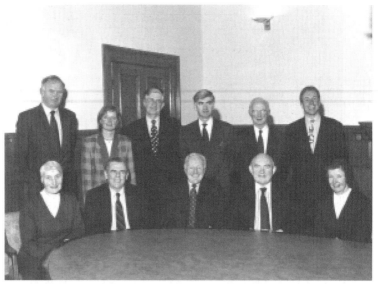

*The first Slowey Board— (front, left to right) Sr Marie McKenna, Donal O'Mahony, Brian Slowey, Chairman, Dr John G. Cooney, Sr Bernadette McMahon;(back, left to right) Michael Jacob, consultant to the Board, Ethel McKenna, Secretary to the Board, Padraic White, Derry O'Donovan, Kevin O'Donnell, Robert Martin, Chief Executive. Absent were M. Doherty and Sr Catherine Mulligan.*

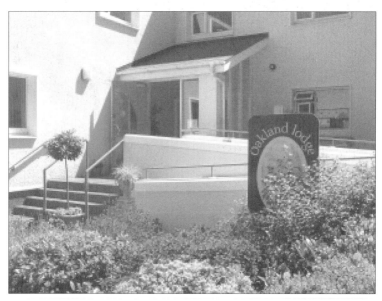

*With the help of the Friends of St Luke's, the redevelopment of the old nurses' home into a hostel for patients and families began in 1995; the name Oakland Lodge was adopted on the suggestion of Eileen Maher, Director of Nursing, in 1996 and the latest extension was opened in May 2005 by Mary Harney, Minister for Health and Children.*

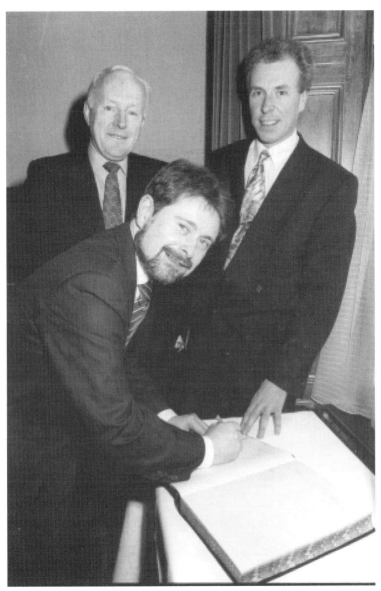

*Minister for Health Brendan Howlin signs the visitors' book while Brian Slowey, Chairman (left) and Robert Martin, Chief Executive, look on.*

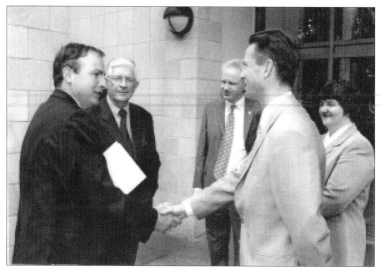

*July 2001: Micheál Martin, Minister for Health and Children, is greeted by (left to right) Padraic White, Chairman, Lorcan Birthistle, Chief Executive, Dr John Armstrong and Eileen Maher, Director of Nursing*

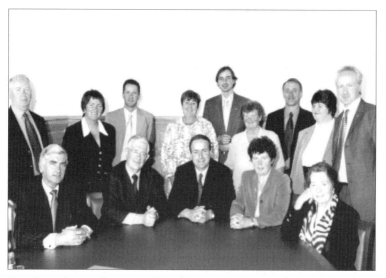

*Board members and senior staff on the occasion of Minister Micheál Martin's visit—(front, left to right) Derry O'Donovan, Padraic White, Chairman, the Minister, Dr Claire MacNicholas, Noreen Slattery; (back, left to right) Liam Dunbar, Mary Courtney, Dr John Armstrong, Louise Richardson, Barry Dempsey, Dr Brendan McLean, Eileen Maher, Lorcan Birthistle*

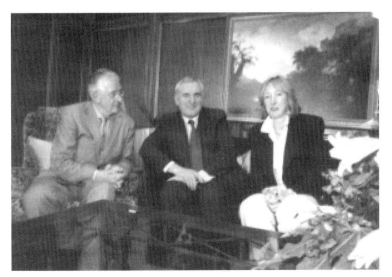

*In June 2002 An Taoiseach Bertie Ahern visited the hospital to open the Patricia Harty Room for patient rest and relaxation. (Left to right) Chairman Padraic White, An Taoiseach, Patricia Harty, Joint Managing Editor of the* Irish Voice, *New York.*

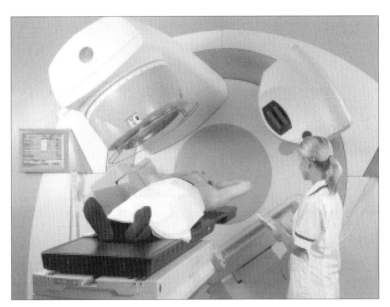

*Installed in 2006, this Linac has a built-in CT scanner, enabling the tumour to be tracked while the radiation is in progress*

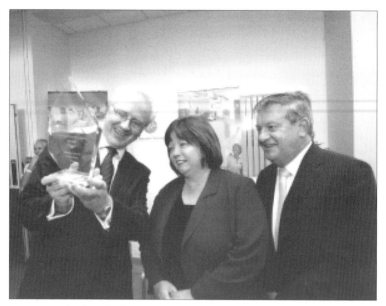

*Lorcan Birthistle, Chief Executive, Mary Harney, Minister for Health and Children, and Stephen McMahon,Chairman of the Irish Patients' Association at the presentation on 7 September 2006 on achieving the highest score of any acute hospital in the country in the 2nd Acute Hospital Hygiene Audit.*

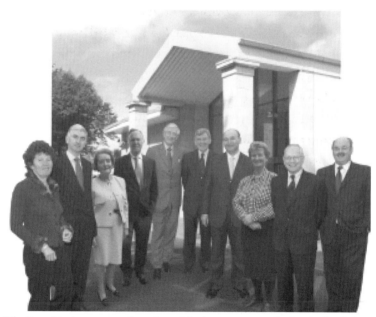

*The Board in late 2004, picured outside the entrance to the hospital—(left to right) Dr Claire MacNicholas, Derry O'Donovan, Noreen Slattery, Eugene Murray, Padraic White, Chairman, Prof. Derry Shanley, John McCormack, Dr Sheelagh Ryan, Prof. Muiris Fitzgerald and Chris Flood*

# Chapter 5: Being a cancer patient

Although people were very afraid of cancer, and with reason, the feeling in Ireland never amounted to the kind of 'cancer-phobia' that was such a strong force in the United States. Ireland was a less media-driven society than the United States so the approach to cancer was more muted. However, no doubt at least partially influenced by the US debate, in 1963 a small group of Irish people decided to act. An immediate catalyst was Dr Austin Darragh's realisation that 100 Irish people every year were dying from one of the most curable forms of the disease, non-melanoma skin cancer[1] (out of a total of slightly fewer than 5,000 cancer deaths a year). As Dr Darragh said later: 'These cancers were visible and 100 per cent curable. It was terrible to realise that those 100 people a year in Ireland died merely because they did not know what to do.' The group first talked to Oliver Chance, and 'thanks to his wisdom and diplomacy' two groups known to him, one anxious to help to raise funds for the hospital, the other committed to improving the level of knowledge about cancer in the community, were advised to pool their resources as one organisation. Thus in 1963 was founded the Conquer Cancer Campaign, later to be called the Irish Cancer Society.

Among the early fundraising people involved were Joe Donoghue and Eric Webb. They joined with Lady Antonia Beckwith, Fred O'Donovan, Drs Dillon Rigby and Jack O'Riordan to form the campaign, whose first chief executive was Frank Doherty. More than forty years later this seems to have been a wholly admirable idea, especially when the fund-raising activities were focused by the inspired borrowing years later from North America of the 'Daffodil Day' concept by Charles Cully. In the Dáil, however, the authoritarian instinct of the day resulted in questions. Minister MacEntee was asked by William Norton of the Labour Party whether he thought it 'desirable that a group of private citizens should be allowed to constitute themselves into a committee for raising money for the purpose of dealing with such a fundamental problem?'[2] What supervision, Norton wanted to know, did the Minister propose to establish over this body? MacEntee took the lofty view that he did not propose to interfere with 'what appears to be public-spirited activity'. He declared that he 'liked to see our citizens displaying initiative.' Noel Browne took a darker view, arguing that the existence of the group suggested 'a very grave reflection on the Minister's efforts to deal with this serious problem.'

Despite a growing awareness of the importance of cancer, it was clear at the same time that the wider ambitions of the Cancer Association were no longer going on the agenda. The new Board of St Luke's accepted the narrow Department of Health view of its function and decided to concentrate its energies on the internal problems of running the hospital. So, despite the help that Oliver Chance had given to the campaign in the early days, in January 1968 the Board decided, after meeting representatives of the Conquer Cancer Campaign, that at least for the moment it would not cooperate with 'bodies collecting monies'. (The hospital changed this policy in a few years, initiating the Friends and engaging fully with the Irish Cancer Society.) When RTÉ broadcast a programme about cancer in 1974 'it was unanimously agreed that the two appearances by the Medical Director recently in the *Tangents* programme, even though anonymous, should for more than one reason not be used for publicity purposes by the Irish Cancer Society and further that RTÉ should be advised accordingly.'

In March 1968 the Board agreed that the idea of amalgamation with St Anne's should no longer be pursued, and in January 1969, citing lack of cooperation from GPs, the Irish Cancer Registry, which had been started in 1957, was wound up. On the other hand, the ever-innovative John Healy in St Luke's began to develop a specialist service based on new French discoveries for acute leukaemia patients. At one time there were more such patients going through St Luke's than through the Royal Marsden in London. The connection with the Paris clinic had been established by Healy, and remained close, even to the extent of flying blood slides from St Luke's patients to be examined in Paris. This service operated in a slightly make-shift way, courtesy of Aer Lingus pilots who used to carry the slides in their pockets. After a while, however, to Healy's dismay, the Board decided that St Luke's should not provide this service any more, and the patients were passed on to St James's.

An *Annual Report* for one of the last years of Oliver Chance's period as Medical Director of St Luke's shows the hospital running with full sail.[3] There had been nearly 2,700 in-patients in the hospital during 1966 and 20,000 out-patients. In addition, country clinics had been conducted in Donegal, Letterkenny, Ballinasloe, Tralee, Limerick, Castlebar, Sligo, Waterford, Athlone and Mullingar. In all, nearly 6,000 patients had been seen in these clinics. St Agatha's, the unit in Cork, conducted clinics virtually every working day, and had over 1,600 patients on its books. The cobalt machine was now up and running in Dublin, and in 1966 treated just under 500 patients in nearly 7,000 sessions. Deep x-ray and contact x-ray patients attended for almost 8,700 sessions. An active department specialised in exploratory tests using various radioactive isotopes including cobalt, (vitamin B12 absorption studies), iodine (for thyroid disorders) and phosphorus (location of eye disorders). In-patients came from all over the country (only one from Northern Ireland); spending a fortnight or so in the wards during the year were 273 patients from Mayo, 315 from Donegal, 252 from Kerry and 109 from Waterford.

The Board of St Luke's was quite small and for twelve years from 1964 to 1976 consisted of a core of Owen Hargadon, the Chairman, Reggie Redmond and Dr Malachy Powell. Mrs Jane Dowdall served from 1968 to her death in 1974, John O'Mahony from 1964 to 1970 and Professor O'Sullivan from 1964 to 1975. They had originally been appointed in 1964 by Seán MacEntee and their appointments had been renewed in 1968 and in 1972. In 1976 a series of new appointments by Labour Minister for Health Brendan Corish included the former Secretary-Registrar Liam Egan and, importantly, Bryan Alton, a gastroenterologist based in the Mater. Dr Alton, who was President of the Royal College of Physicians at the time, had especially wide contacts among the Fianna Fáil élite.

In marked contrast to the present method of management, the Board was closely involved in the day-to-day running of the hospital. The Secretary-Registrar Liam Egan retired in October 1973 and was replaced by Esther Byrne, who had been the Assistant Secretary. Neither saw themselves as a 'chief executive' in the modern sense. The full Board met once a month, and the hospital committee (a subset of the board) met once a fortnight (23 times a year) to discuss detailed management questions. Many of the staff reported directly to the Board. Here, for instance, is 'Matron requesting permission for Staff Nurse Maura Coughlan to attend a course at the College of Commerce, Rathmines for 1 week at a cost of £15. Read, noted and approved'.[4]

The committee was very much hands-on. Every fortnight they checked the reconciliation of the three bank accounts, signed some 200 cheques and authorised unrecoverable debts e.g. account 70/ 328 'agreed to write off the sum of £7.35'. Appointments and resignations were noted, requests for unpaid leave approved, pensions and ex-gratia payments made, for everyone from consultants to temporary assistant gardeners. Requisitions of all sorts were examined: in November 1973, for instance, the committee approved the purchase of an image intensifier on the advice of the chief physicist for £7,000; and bought three books for the library, a dictaphone and a chain block hoist.

Members of the Board could often be seen about the hospital, for example, Breda Carroll (former Chief Medical Laboratory Technologist) remembers Reggie Redmond popping into her lab one day to enquire: 'How are you getting on? Did you get that computer yet?'[5] To her, the modern style, when the Board comes only as a formal entourage 'is almost like a return to the formality of the old days'.

*Working in St Luke's*

Kathleen (Kay) Rochford, who became Secretary-Manager of the hospital in 1983, joined the accounts department in 1956. Working in the old house, she remembers the fine ceiling, with 'cherubs flying over us all day', and the silk tapestry on the walls. The staff would gather in the appropriate dining room for their 1 shilling lunch (with complimentary beverages). There was, as Josephine Fitzmaurice remembered, a strict hierarchy: there were two separate rooms in the canteen—the main big dining room was for nursing staff and clerical staff; the sisters, radiographers and physicists sat elsewhere. The consultants, the Matron, the Medical Director and the Secretary-Manager all had their specific seats in the middle of the room. The ward sisters had a special room for their coffee and fresh toast of a morning. Yet another separate room was set aside for the porters to have their meals. 'The divisions seem extraordinary now, but at the time it was normal; we didn't think anything to it and we didn't feel badly about it.'

The social life is fondly remembered. Every Christmas 'we would enjoy a great Christmas party which was a black tie event arranged by the Board through Matron Mary Dixon who issued the invitations for our partners who would arrive after the staff dinner. We would then proceed to the nurses' home with our guests and dance and party until the early hours.' Permission for these events on hospital premises was duly sought from the hospital committee; in April 1974, for example, a letter from the staff social committee 'requesting permission to hold the finals of the table tennis competition in the nuses' home on 24 April' was read and approved.[6]

In the early 1970s the newly-joined radiologist Michael Moriarty had suggested to Liam Egan that a social committee be established to organise events during the year. This was a great success, and no doubt significantly developed the strong esprit de corps that was a feature of the hospital. To 21st-century eyes there is something admirable, but perhaps a little old-fashioned, about the staff's willingness to take part in so many activities. This degree of after-hours involvement is certainly not a feature of the modern hospital. Kay Rochford recalls 'arrangements were made for soirées, dances, beagling with the Curragh Beagles on Sundays; we travelled on the canal at Robertstown and dined in a local hotel. We had a trip to Athlone and cruised on the Shannon; treasure hunts on Saturdays were great fun; fancy dress dances and concerts tested the talents of the staff—one of our porters arranged for us to go to Athy to dine and dance—oh for the days when we all had such energy!' There was even, in the 1980s, courtesy of Dr Michael Maher, a staff greyhound, the woefully misnamed 'Highfield Flier'. His upkeep and training fees were deducted from the wages of participants.

To the outside world St Luke's remained a mysterious, not to say sinister place. Lorcan Birthistle, Chief Executive from 2001 to late 2007, grew up in the neighbourhood and remembers that he and his friends would not hesitate to trespass in neighbouring gardens, but would never enter the grounds of St Luke's. He vividly remembers also the patients walking into Rathgar for a drink or for small purchases, some in their slippers, many marked with purple lines on their heads and necks—aiming marks for the radiotherapy, which is now done on a mask.

In one of his books John McGahern describes how his hero visits a ward where his aunt lies dying. He arrives by taxi: 'We turned in at the hospital gates, with its two white globes on the piers; the city gave way to trees and soft fields and suddenly in the middle of the fields the concrete and glass block of the hospital rose like some rock'. The aunt is in a bad way: 'The pain's still there,' she says, 'God and the brandy is all that's any use now. It's all I get any value out of.'

Later the hero visits the hospital one evening, accompanied by his nurse girl-friend, and creates a vivid picture of the long wards divided by glass half-walls, at night.

> We climbed the bare concrete stairs and went through swing doors. Suddenly we were in a long hall with beds on either side. The ward was in darkness, except for the lines of moonlight, and the blue light beside the night nurse sitting behind the glass at the other end . . . in the dim light I stood and listened to the far roar of the night traffic through the city. I thought I heard a moan or few words of prayer in the night, but could not be certain because of my pounding heart. All were women in this ward and they all had cancer. [7]

The story ends sadly: 'I won't be coming back [to St Luke's]' says John McGahern's fictional aunt, 'I've fought long enough and hard enough and it's beaten me, bad luck to it.'[8]

For the patients, as we have seen, there was relief in the fact that nearly everyone in the hospital either had cancer or was not afraid to look it in the eye. (There would always be some non-cancers being treated with radiation, and these relatively healthy patients diluted the mix somewhat.) Indeed the story is told of a patient coming timidly into the ward and, as he put it, 'I saw fellas there who were much worse off than me, and though I shouldn't say it, I was delighted!' This freedom from constraint, combined with the devoted nursing and the wooded, almost rural surroundings, generally made the stay in St Luke's a positive experience. Dr John Healy remembers several patients at the outside clinics saying to him 'that was the only holiday I ever had'.

Michael O'Halloran was regularly renewed as chair of the medical staff committee until August 1973 when he was finally appointed Medical Director. As such he took the view, in common with the Board and most of the medical environment, that the hospital's function was simply to provide a radiation therapy service when required to the Irish hospital system.[9] He was a very different man from Oliver Chance whose vision of a national cancer centre of excellence had driven the hospital in its early days. O'Halloran was not inclined to proselytise the benefits of radiotherapy or particularly to 'market' the hospital's service. As a friend of Michael O'Halloran's, Bryan Alton is believed to have been an important influence in persuading the latter to support Des Carney's joint appointment as medical oncologist to St Luke's and the Mater.

Dr James Fennelly was the country's first medical oncologist, based in St Vincent's, just after its move to Elm Park, though the fact that his first allocated beds were in the hospice at Harold's Cross hardly amounted to a ringing endorsement. Nonetheless, his work was beginning to attract attention. Reggie Redmond recalls meeting Oliver Chance in Grafton Street in the early 1970s and Chance telling him that the discipline he had devoted his life to was no longer of great importance, and that chemotherapy was the way of the future. Throughout the hospital's history there has been a periodically recurring awareness that, however well aimed and titrated, radiation therapy is ultimately a burning of malignant cells, and it would be better if something less crude were available—and that the 'something better' was just on the horizon. For St Luke's the consequence was that at a time when some in the medical profession were beginning to doubt the long-term utility of radiation, the relatively modest approach adopted by the Medical Director and the Board contributed to changing St Luke's from a central voice in the treatment of cancer to a specialist unit, somewhat off the beaten track.

In 1972 a new Board was appointed by Erskine Childers (later, briefly, President of Ireland), and more or less the same group settled down to their third four-year term of running the hospital. Economic conditions were set to get increasingly tough. The first shock came in 1973 when the Arab oil-producing countries, as a manoeuvre in the Arab-Israeli conflict, effectively quadrupled the price of oil. Since Ireland was largely dependant both on imported energy and export sales to countries equally struck by this blow, the public finances reeled. It was very soon after this that the hospital was obliged to request the Department of Health to authorise its first overdraft, of £50,000. Four years later this leapt to £250,000.

The economic stringency forced a number of unpalatable decisions. One, which had considerable long-term effects, was to refuse a proposal to turn one of the private rooms into a post-operative intensive care ward. Post-operative care had been a feature of St Luke's. The very big operations necessitated by an attempt to remove largely affected areas of the body left patients extremely weak and vulnerable. As the techniques of post-operative intensive care evolved Dr Margaret Gallagher in particular became skilled; so much so that surgeons were attracted to work in St Luke's, knowing that post-operative work, normally assigned to junior doctors not long qualified, would be in specialised hands. The effect of the decision not to augment the intensive care capability was to limit the hospital's ability to provide a complete cancer service of surgery, radiation and chemotherapy. Surgery is still in 2007 the preferred treatment for about half of cancer patients, typically those whose cancer remains local rather than metastasised. However, as the equipment required for a fully-functioning theatre became more sophisticated and expensive, the hospital's financial problems meant that investment in theatre equipment was not maintained. As the Director of Nursing,

Eileen Maher, remembers, when she first came to the hospital in 1995 the theatre lamp had been acquired second-hand from the Mater, and was doubtfully reliable. The practice of surgery in the hospital steadily declined.

By bad luck the oil shocks occurred at almost exactly the time when the hospital started to seek quotations and support for the so-called linear accelerator (commonly called the 'Linac'). At this time the hospital's radiotherapy equipment consisted of a 300 kV Siemens unit, two 200kV x-ray machines and a low voltage x-ray machine for skin cancers; the first cobalt bomb had been joined by a second in 1966, and another based in St Agatha's in Cork. Radium was in use for inter-cavity and interstitial treatments using a method pioneered in the Manchester Christie Hospital.

## The Physics Department

The central service unit for all this equipment was the Physics Department. Its core function was to control and maintain the often unwieldy and un-biddable, yet still lethal, radioactive sources to produce curative doses for patients; their use of pure science in this way was a departure from normal hospital practice.

The Chief Physicist, John O'Connor, had been the first full-time hospital physicist in the country when in 1949, aged twenty-five, he joined St Anne's from University College Dublin. In 1952 he was one of those involved in the exodus from Ranelagh to Rathgar, when he moved to Oakland to set up the new department in St Luke's. His work at this time resulted in a number of seminal papers on dosimetry and the so-called 'O'Connor density scaling theorem' which are still essential texts in the field.

By 1969 the unit employed three physicists and eight technicians who between them serviced the two cobalt machines, six other x-ray machines and the active 'isotope department'. One of these machines, the Muller 200 kV rotation therapy unit, had soaked up a good deal of physicists' time—it had presented, as John O'Connor put it in a report to the *Bulletin of the Hospital Physicists Association,* 'unfamiliar and formidable problems of dosimetry'. The Muller was now 'in honourable retirement, its functions having been largely taken over by the two cobalt units'. O'Connor recorded that the radiotherapy department treated 2,500 patients a year and the nuclear medicine facility carried out over 3,000 tests.[10]

Supporting all this activity were the mechanical and electronic workshops associated with the department. John O'Connor was a firm believer in the value of a good workshop—indeed the almost experimental nature of the equipment made this essential. There were no neat manuals and few textbooks. As well as maintaining the equipment, often on low budgets, the staff devised special devices to make handling the radioactive materials safe, and jigs and shields for individual patients. The constant pressure from the clinicians was for more penetrating power to access deep-seated tumours, and more precision to target them. The problem was complicated by the fact that inside the body tumours are not fixed like bone, but are living, shifting entities, changing shape with the patient's posture, like a restless sleeper's breast or stomach.

The machines the manufacturers produced could deliver the force, but it was always up to the individual hospitals to calibrate and control them—just as a bicycle manufacturer relies on the purchaser to learn how to ride, or the computer manufacturer expects the user to learn how to use the machine. Partly this was because the manufacturers themselves generally had non-medical backgrounds—the supplier of the hospital's first cobalt machine was the subsidiary of a railway engineering firm. As much as six months was taken by the Physics Department in St Luke's between the time this machine was installed and when it was ready to treat patients.

The calibration technique used was to measure output in the flexible medium of water, and then to convert these measurements to human tissue. Sam McKenzie in the workshop built a water tank inside which was an ion chamber (recording the beam values) that moved through the tank in three dimensions with steel cables that moved an indicator outside the room. The controls were precise to fractions of a millimetre. As David Murnaghan, later Chief Physicist at St Luke's, put it: 'You looked for places with the same dose of radiation and every time you found it you marked it on a piece of paper.' Part of John O'Connor's international reputation derived from the papers he wrote to enable water-based measurements to be converted to tissue, lungs and bones. After months of work full iso-dose maps were produced for the clinicians.

A different problem was encountered sometime later when the first Linac was delivered. The beam had a tendency to 'drift', which often meant that it had to be recalibrated. There was much discussion of this in the technical journals. In St Luke's workshop Eric Feeney built a series of attached devices that monitored the beam constantly, so adjustments could be made on the spot. Similar devices are now standard on all third-generation Linacs.

In these early days, although there was sharing of techniques and ideas through journals and meetings, each hospital created its own systems and controls responding to local conditions. The Holt Christie version of St Luke's water tank, for instance, was made out of old bomber plane parts. The ingenuity of the workshop often kept machines going that in a better economic climate would have been replaced.

### National Radiation Monitoring Service

The presence on the St Luke's campus of the National Radiation Monitoring Service was a constant reminder of the dangers inherent in working with such materials. The first generation of radiation workers had seriously underestimated those dangers, and there were numerous fatalities as a result. By the 1920s, however, international agreement had been reached on the basic principles of radiation protection. When St Luke's was founded, therefore, there were well-understood protocols aimed at protecting those working the machines every day, plus, of course, the patients and the public. For the staff a system of film badges was established, using a design from the Holt Christie Hospital in Manchester. These badges contained a strip of photographic film covered by various filters (metal, plastic etc.) which enabled laboratory staff to identify the type of radiation (alpha, beta, x-ray etc.) that the wearer had been exposed to, and by the darkening of the film by how much. The system ensured that cumulative doses did not exceed recommended levels. Since St Luke's was using more radiation than anywhere else in the country, quite soon the hospital was providing a film badge service for x-ray staff in other hospitals. In 1963 the service was formally named the National Radiation Monitoring Service (NRMS).

In the 1970s this monitoring service was extended also to university laboratories and industrial plants, such as paper manufacturers, who used radiation in level and thickness gauges. By 1975 the service was handling 31,500 badges every year. As David Murnaghan recalls, it was very rare, 'that anything serious emerged' though he remembers one case when a nurse's badge was returned extremely black. Alarm bells rang immediately, but it turned out that a patient had lost the cord to his pyjamas, and the nurse had used the safety pin on the badge to hold his trousers up while he was receiving his treatment. The story neatly illustrates the difference between the low day-in-day-out dose acceptable for staff and the much higher tumour-killing dose given for a limited time to patients.

As the largest user in the country, the hospital became recognised as the expert resource for matters to do with radiation, for instance in assessing the amount of radioactivity in the Irish Sea. The presence of Windscale/Sellafield across the water made this a sensitive political issue. After the fire in the plant in 1957, although no one died and the epidemiological effect was untraceable, there was continuous concern about contamination from across the sea. Samples would be collected from Carlingford to Wexford and analysed in the NRMS. Despite the paranoia, the NRMS found that its results correlated very closely to those published by the British Department of Agriculture and Fisheries. In response to professional and public concern the government commissioned a study by Bernadette Herity of UCD and St Luke's and colleagues of the incidence of childhood leukaemia (acute lymphoblastic leukaemia) and other lymphoid malignancies. The study, which was published in 1986, failed to identify any cause for concern, showing that the rates of disease were the same for coastal as inland districts, apart from a small unexplained excess mortality in a three-mile strip of the east coast in the period 1974–6.

The badges were only part of the scheme of staff protection. Over the years St Luke's had built up considerable practical experience in making safe high-energy x-ray and gamma ray installations.

The cobalt bombs, for instance, emitted penetrating gamma rays at such an intensity that immensely thick walls of high density concrete were required. To enable medical staff to oversee patients during treatment the observation windows had to provide the same degree of safety, so special fittings had to be designed. Nowadays the same effect is achieved by closed circuit television. The protection of patients was a major concern. The equipment, as we have seen, needed constant attention to ensure that the right dose was delivered to the right spot. To ensure as little skin exposure as possible when treating deeply seated tumours, for instance, rotating beams were used that could move round the target.

The 1973 energy crisis stimulated the government to look more seriously at ways of extending its electricity generation. They set up a Nuclear Energy Board with a brief to advise on the practicalities of setting up a nuclear power station on the site the ESB had identified at Carnsore Point in County Wexford. John O'Connor was on the board of the NEB, and for some years, since the NEB did not have a laboratory, it and the NRMS operated on parallel tracks, supplementing each other's services. In 1979 the Three Mile Island accident galvanised public opinion against the proposal, and a series of colourful protests combined with intensive lobbying persuaded the government to back away.[11] The project was formally abandoned in 1981, and a generation later a wind farm was built on the site. Subsequently the NEB absorbed the activities of the NRMS, taking with them some staff from St Luke's.[12]

### The first linear accelerator

The saga of the first Linac (the hospital now has eight) was to run throughout the 1970s. This was a much more sophisticated and expensive device than the previous purchase, the cobalt unit, producing a more precise beam of energy targetable at deep tumours. The linear accelerator is not based on natural radiation like radium or cobalt, but uses microwave technology to create high-energy x-rays that are shaped to form a beam that matches the patient's tumor. Years before, John O'Connor had considered and rejected these machines, which were then in their early years of development, on grounds of costs and their experimental nature. Now they were becoming almost standard equipment, and the first quotations were sought in June 1973, but the Department of Health sat on the request for approval. In August 1974 the Board was told that difficulties and breakdowns in the old cobalt machines were requiring patients to be treated at abnormal hours and this was causing staffing difficulties. The Board wrote to the Department in October and again in November asking for a decision. It was not until two years later, in May 1976, that the contract for a building to house the Linac was signed. The machine was finally delivered in 1978, and the unit was formally opened in November 1979 by the then Minister, Charles Haughey.

*Fear and euphemism*

Although in the 1970s much more was written and broadcast about cancer than before, some at least of the patients and their families were quite vague as to what ailed them. Breda Carroll, who joined the lab in 1976, remembers being accosted on her way into work by anxious visitors enquiring: 'What kind of hospital is this?', a question which required a tactfully evasive answer. However kind and straightforward the clinician might be, the diagnosis was intensely frightening, and any patient might be forgiven for reacting as Janette Byrne did when told in the elaborate 21st-century manner of her tumour: 'fading words now, making no sense, "Blah, blah, blah . . ." I shake my head . . . No! No! No! The tears are flowing.'[13] Catholic education taught that the last days enduring cancer were more than simply being exposed to a painful disease—they were a test. As Seán Feehan wrote, in the context of his wife's death from breast cancer:

> Suffering is the most merciless of realities, yet without it our lives cannot be complete. It is the thermometer of one's character. It strips one down to the very bone. It can make the average man go under, the egoist become still more egotistical, the hard of heart still more cruel, the small mind become more treacherous and mean. But it is not suffering so much that matters as [much as] the way we bear it. Suffering is powerless to destroy those great and noble spirits who have expurgated all self-love from their lives.[14]

No wonder that many shrank from diagnosis, like the elderly aunt in one of Francis Brett Young's medical novels, who modestly resisted having her sore breast examined by the new young doctor for so long that by the time the diagnosis was made, it was far too late to do anything. So great was the fear that doctors resisted using the plain words. Dr John Healy recalls that he never used the word 'cancer' in discussion with patients, referring merely to 'a little growth' or some similar euphemism. Dr O'Halloran similarly avoided the word. This was not an exclusively Irish phenomenon; a study in the 1960s suggested that as many as 90 per cent of American physicians did not tell patients of a cancer diagnosis, and Alexander Solzenitsyn recalled from his days in the cancer ward in Tashkent in the 1950s how the doctors fenced around everything they said. In her vivid account of her last days suffering from breast and brain tumours, Ruth Picardie commented that 'cancer is steeped with fear and euphemism'—both in and beside the patients' beds. To counter this universal emotion, a soothing babble of technical terms is used everywhere—the specialists are not cancer doctors, they are oncologists; they talk of 'growths', 'neoplasms' and 'malignancies' being 'advanced', 'progressing' (is that good?) or 'secondary', surgery is 'successful' (but that does not necessarily mean the patient is cured) and they discuss 'management' and 'palliation'.[15]

In the days before the Internet, patients were expected to be docile and accepting of medical authority. Information was not easily acquired; patients were discouraged from accessing textbooks and other references.[16] The purpose of this obfuscation was to sustain the patient's morale. Yet there is little scientific evidence that a good attitude is conducive to cure. Indeed Professor John Crown, a consultant at St Luke's, has robustly dismissed the notion that a strong will to live makes any difference to the outcome.[17] On the other hand, cancer is a life-threatening and life-changing disease. Almost everyone dealing with cancer patients puts great stress on establishing coping mechanisms 'to combine mental healing with physical healing' as St Luke's Director of Nursing Eileen Maher puts it. As Dr Healy commented 'the atmosphere in the hospital is hugely important.' The nursing staff are of course crucial to this, and as Dr Healy remembers, the first Matron Mary Dixon was 'a very fine woman' who set extremely high standards of care and cleanliness in the hospital.

*Research*

Another important activity on the St Luke's campus was research. When the first cobalt unit was finally opened in 1963, the Minister had commented especially on the growth of research in St Luke's, led by the Professor of Pathology in TCD, R. A. Q. O'Meara. With the usual optimism of such moments, Seán MacEntee noted that research workers all over the world were engaged in work 'that would make the conquest of cancer more certain'. One such team was Professor O'Meara's; and though he was anxious to avoid undue optimism he could report beneficial results in selected cases. The Minister wished the Professor every success and, speaking as an ex-Minister for Finance, noted carefully that the research 'has been conducted without recourse to public funds'.

As the world knows, the 'conquest of cancer' is still to seek. On the other hand, a steady stream of research papers has been emanating from St Luke's to this day. Although nowadays such active intellectual interest is customary, even obligatory, in the 1960s this was by no means so. In 1970 Professor O'Meara described the ongoing research, which was largely concerned with the way tumours inter-reacted with the surrounding normal cells. [18] His own great discovery in this field was made in 1957 after a two-year programme into how tumours grow and spread. He identified that the threads of fibrin commonly seen around tumours were not, as had been thought, part of the body's defence against the tumour, but on the contrary were part of the way tumours established themselves.

However, despite the enormous amount of work, by Professor O'Meara at St Luke's among others, scientists were still more or less in the dark about cancer. They could distinguish the ragged malignant cells from healthy ones under the microscope, but knew almost nothing knew about what was happening inside them. There was even considerable pessimism about whether science would ever be able to penetrate the mysteries of the cell. Sir Macfarlane Burnett, the Nobel prize-winning immunologist, declared in the mid-1970s that 'so far there has been no human benefit whatever from all that has been learned from molecular biology' and the science journalist June Goodfield confirmed in her 1975 book *Cancer under siege*: 'There is very little that we can yet do or are likely to be able to do concerning a basic change in the internal genetics of the cell.'[19] Happily, this was too pessimistic. A series of astonishing discoveries in molecular biology at the end of the 1970s and the beginning of the 1980s was for the very first time to cut through the confusion about the true nature of cancer.

# Chapter 6: A marriage made in the Department

In the late 1970s and early 1980s certain key discoveries about the mechanisms of the cell made it seem that the long and frustrating search for the inner nature of cancer was nearly over. Unfortunately, time has shown that the full mystery of cancer still has many twists. Nonetheless, in these exciting years cancer was definitively identified as a corruption in the DNA (genetic component) of the cell. This was an important step. Although fat cells, brain cells, blood cells, bone cells and muscle cells seem as different as can be, they are all controlled at heart by the expression of the same set of genes, working at the speed of an electric circuit. Like a kind of sophisticated Morse code, these genes consist of long chains of just four chemical bases—adenine (A), cytosine (C), guanine (G) and thymine (T)—in various orders. A typical gene has several thousand such bases which, when combined, instruct other parts of the cell to this or that activity. Astonishingly, it seemed that a mutation initiating cancer might consist of an error in only one.

Every human has trillions of cells. They are, mostly, vanishingly small for such important determiners of health. Cells in their hundreds of thousands are typically organised into cooperative assemblies called tissues (skin, bone, nerves, muscles etc) which are connected by protein-based materials. Perhaps the most remarkable of these proteins is collagen, a long, stiff, rope-like protein which forms the basis of skin and bone. All the activities in creating and renewing tissues are controlled by the long strings of DNA in the heart of each cell. Cancer is basically started by a series of mistakes in this manual, driving the cell to act out of character. There are many different types of such malfunction, and in the late 1970s it was discovered that cancers require more than one mutation before they evolve into full-blown tumours.

A practical result of the long path to full-blown cancer is that, like early pregnancies that miscarry, nature may not allow things to develop so far. We know very little about these early pre-cancers, and why so-called benign growths fail to develop the fatal ability to metastasise. The cancers that we are conscious of are generally those that have progressed a long way—as if the first anyone knew of a baby was when it suddenly appeared from the womb. Monitoring of cervical cancer by smear tests demonstrated this. The smear test enabled doctors to identify cells that had just begun their journey towards full malignancy; and by no means all would actually get there. A 1991 study of cancer in Ireland confirmed that 'many of the abnormalities, even the serious ones, will disappear in time without any treatment and it is not possible at present to distinguish between the serious pre-cancerous condition and that which will not progress.'[1]

While the molecular scientists opened up more and more of the secrets of the cell, in 1981 the veteran campaigner Richard Doll (with his colleague Richard Peto) produced an influential analysis of the incidence of cancer in *The causes of cancer*.[2] This was an attempt to develop his critical association of lung cancer and tobacco use to all cancers. Of course, without a detailed understanding of what cancer is and how it originates, these kinds of studies often raise more questions than they answer. What are we to conclude from the fact that the age-adjusted breast cancer rate in England was, according to Doll and Peto's figures, twice that in Spain? Or that stomach cancers were twice as common in Italy as in France?[3] In due course it may be that we will understand exactly why there are such wild differences between the incidence across the world of different cancers. There was, for instance, a 200 times difference between the skin cancer rates in Queensland, Australia and Mumbai in India, and we can assume that this has something to do with exposure to sun. But is the key factor the genetic inheritance (including, but by no means limited to, skin colour) or the relative propensity to go out into the noonday sun? Or these combined with something else altogether, for instance the proportion of meat in the diet? Imaginative answers to such questions are either the start of science or the stimulus for quackery, depending on taste.

Using US statistics, Doll and Peto claimed that as many as 80 per cent of cancers were 'avoidable'—if only people were to adopt likely or socially acceptable methods. Diet and tobacco use, which they considered contributed to perhaps two-thirds of cancers, could theoretically be controlled. But although they believed that obliging women to get pregnant by fifteen years of age (and thereafter their husbands and they to remain strictly monogamous) would significantly reduce breast and uterine cancer rates, they had to admit that such a law was not at all likely.

*Proportion of cancer deaths attributable to various factors*

| | |
|---|---|
| Diet | 35% |
| Tobacco | 30% |
| Infection | 10% |
| Reproductive and sexual behaviour | 7% |
| Occupation | 4% |
| Geophysical factors | 3% |
| Alcohol | 3% |
| Pollution | 2% |
| Food additives | 1% |
| Industrial products | 1% |
| Medicines and medical procedures | 1% |
| Unknown | 6% |
| *Total US cancer deaths* | *100%* |

*Source*: R. Doll and R. Peto 1981

For the staff of St Luke's these insights had little immediate clinical significance. Just as it took two generations after Koch's discovery of mycobacteria tuberculosis for a cure to emerge, this dawning knowledge of the deep causes of cancer was slow to produce cures. (To speed this process, a new discipline called 'translation studies' has been established to accelerate the transfer of knowledge from laboratory to clinic and back again.) None of the techniques in use, whether chemotherapy, radiotherapy or surgery, could distinguish a malignant from a healthy cell, and certainly none could discriminate to the level of the individual cell where the mutation was occurring. They were sledgehammers used to crack nuts. Although they became increasingly sophisticated as time wore on, it was ultimately a tribute to the marvellous resilience of the human body that they worked so often.

### A new Board

In May 1980 the long-serving Chairman of St Luke's, Owen Hargadon, retired from the civil service and from the Board. He was replaced by Reggie Redmond, who was to lead the hospital through the troubled 1980s. He took the helm at the beginning of a hectic decade in Irish political life. Two factors loomed over the local scene.

The first was the enormous public debt built up by the Fianna Fáil government of 1977 to 1981 in their ill-considered 'boom and bloom' budget. The second was the divisive figure of Charles Haughey. Haughey had triumphed over the deep and lasting divisions inside the Fianna Fáil party to become leader and Taoiseach in 1979. His early promise to tighten belts and subdue the out-of-control public finances was not fulfilled, and crowd-pleasing gestures raised average pay rates in the public service by almost 30 per cent in 1980. Another of these gestures was the so-called 'common contract' for consultants, which set in stone Ireland's unique public/private mix of medical service. It was, incidentally, widely believed that Bryan Alton was instrumental in persuading Charles Haughey of the terms. As usual with the Irish medical service the new contract created anomalies and dissension. For many months the hospital's senior consultant, Dr John Healy, refused to sign the contract, and in September 1983 the Board was told that Professor Des Carney, who had clinics in St Luke's and in the Mater, had two common contracts, one from each hospital, and they were different.

By the election in 1981 the national debt was found to have trebled since 1977, and current public spending was up by 50 per cent. This was to set the tone for a series of alternative governments headed by Haughey and Garret FitzGerald—the so-called 'revolving door Taoisigh'—in which control of the public finances was the key political battleground. Unfortunately, coalition government and frequent elections are not conducive to the necessary disciplines of increased taxation and reduced public expenditure. The working through of the effects of a new oil price rise in 1979 did not help matters, nor did the constant violent distractions from the north and the so-called 'GUBU' incidents in the south. In the 1982–6 FitzGerald government the Minister for Health, Barry Desmond, cut public spending on hospitals by 1.5 per cent. This seemed bad at the time, but as Maev-Ann Wren points out: 'Desmond is remembered, in the medical profession in particular, as the man who savaged the health service. In relative terms the charge does not stick. Much worse was to come under the government elected in 1987.'[4]

This was not good news for St Luke's, being at the unfashionable end of cancer treatment, just when an exciting range of computer-driven hi-tech possibilities, both curative and diagnostic, were opening up. As a result, it was one of the new private hospitals, the Mater Private, that initiated MRI scanning in Ireland in 1986, while St Luke's increasingly struggled to maintain its ageing equipment in working order. A further series of cuts in the health service under Rory O'Hanlon between 1987 and 1991 reduced hospital beds by nearly 15 per cent, at a time when new medical regimes and possibilities meant that the numbers of patients treated in hospital rose from 552,000 in 1980 to 647,000 in 1990 (by 2000 the figure was 876,000—a staggering 60 per cent increase in 20 years[5]). Simultaneously health service recruitment was embargoed, and hospital charges were introduced.

The new Board started with an awkward inter-regnum which underlined how low the hospital was on the Department's agenda. The term of office of the Hargadon Board expired in May 1980 and no new Board was formally appointed for four full months. In practice, however, because the Board was so very closely involved with the day-to-day working of the hospital, the remaining members of the old Board felt obliged to soldier on signing cheques and so on without formal authority to do so. Eventually, this had to come to an end. Finally, in late August Reggie Redmond wrote to the Minister, Michael Woods, asking him to stabilise matters. As he put it: 'Some Board members have expressed reservations about the use of the seal by the Board in such circumstances and indeed even our authority to sign cheques has been questioned. These and other necessary decisions made by the board combine to make members generally uneasy.'[6] Very soon after this a new Board consisting of Reggie Redmond (Chairman), Dr Bryan Alton, Sr Columba McNamara, Dr Malachy Powell, Liam Egan, Dermot Flynn and Professor Ciaran McCarthy was appointed for a four-year term.

The minutes of the meetings of this Board, as it laboured through the 1980s, make depressing reading. As early as August 1981 it was noted that the hospital was exceeding its financial allocation; a year later the Department cut its revenue by £160,000—and gave the hospital permission for an overdraft of £500,000. In 1984 the revenue allocation of £4.27 million was £177,000 short of the budget—though, as it happened, by tight control of drugs this was turned into a narrow surplus. From February 1985 only one theatre was to be used, and by May 1986 this was only in operation half of the week (unfortunately the savings that might have resulted from this were diminished by the staff's refusal to transfer to other duties). In May 1987, facing a shortfall of £603,700, the unpalatable decision was made to close one of the wards, with the loss of 36 beds; in theory this was to last only until Christmas, but it was, in effect, permanent. This closure, and the savings effected by a lengthy porters' strike, enabled the hospital to remain in budget for that year.

The close scrutiny of the day-to-day activities of the hospital by the Board and its subset, the hospital committee, continued as before. Not that they were without challenge. In 1981 the new Matron, Margaret Johnston, who is remembered as something of a radical, rebelled against the old-fashioned custom of Matron handing out wages cheques personally to the nurses. Eighteen months later a row broke out about the appointment of a ward sister. Reading between the lines it seems likely that Ms Johnston felt that this appointment should be in her hands, and said so perhaps too bluntly (the Board minutes described her letter as 'grossly insulting and not acceptable in tone or content'). In the circumstances she refused to sit on an interview board, which the Board recorded as 'a point-blank refusal to carry out the instructions of this Board'. The Board resolved to consult its legal advisors. However, nothing happened, and in August 1983 a kind of reconciliation took place, with the Board minuting 'we are willing to start afresh'. Some months after this Mrs McCambridge, as she had become, left the hospital to become Matron and Director of Nursing at the Royal Hospital Donnybrook.

Much detailed work was still done by the hospital committee which continued to meet once a fortnight. On 25 April 1984, for instance, the committee met as usual. The Chairman, Reggie Redmond, sent his apologies, and a wish was recorded that he would soon get better. No cheques were signed, but otherwise the matters discussed were as normal. Requisitions were approved (24 white coats at £15 each, some linoleum for the scanning room floor at £312, five swivel chairs for the medical records office, three bottle racks 'for use with the Heron bedpan washers'). This was not an automatic procedure: David Murnaghan wanted a new filing cabinet, but before giving its approval, the committee wanted to know 'what papers it is proposed to file in this cabinet, as it is not envisaged that there could be a lot of correspondence involved in his position as Radiation Protection Advisor?' (His answer was that he was legally obliged to store some records for as much as twenty years.)

The accountant brought to the committee's attention a large increase in expenditure on drugs. Dr Sabra, the Chief Pharmacist, explained that there was a definite increase in the general usage of chemotherapy and also marked price increases (inflation was 8.6 per cent that year, down from over 10 per cent in 1983). He also reported that two particular drugs for patients had cost £7,000. Other business included approving the Medical Director's suggestion that an extra clinic be held in Sligo in May to catch up with a backlog of patients; payment of relocation expenses for the new medical oncologist Dr Des Carney who was coming to Dublin from the US; and the bank reconciliation had revealed that there was nearly £1,700 in uncashed cheques—the Secretary-Manager was requested to contact staff and creditors and urge them to cash these cheques 'without further delay'.

## A marriage made in the Department

### *The Friends of St Luke's*

One of the first items on the agenda of the main Board was a letter from the Medical Director Michael O'Halloran 'suggesting the establishment of a committee as a fund-raising group under the title of Friends of St Luke's'. This repeated a suggestion originally made in May by Dr Rutledge of the outgoing Board. In January 1981 the idea of the Friends of St Luke's was agreed in principle. This new organisation was to be independent of the Board and run by an outside group. It was finally incorporated and launched in November 1981. The first directors were Michael O'Halloran, Paul O'Neill, Michael Moriarty, Tom Fitzpatrick, James Milton, John Conway and Norman Kearns. Brian Campbell was Company Secretary and first Appeals Director.

Led by Michael O'Halloran's intimate knowledge of the needs of the hospital, the Friends set themselves two initial targets of equipment purchase. The first was a computer-driven simulator, to greatly improve the precision and accuracy of treatment planning, and the second was another Linac. On 1 July 1982 O'Halloran reported on a successful meeting he had had with the Department of Health: 'The Department has agreed to buy a linear accelerator machine for the hospital on the understanding that the Friends will pay for the twin treatment room which is required and is estimated to cost about £0.5m.' The board agreed to this proposal, and sprang into action. The listing of the top 500 companies published in *Irish Business* proved a happy hunting ground, but the bulk of work was done by literally hundreds of groups across the country, most of whom had close experience, as a result of the sickness of relatives or friends, of the hospital's service. The spring 1983 newsletter recorded a total of 89 activities undertaken over the previous six months, ranging from simple collections from, among others, the ballroom staff at the Green Isle Hotel, Rathmines Senior College, and the Post Office staff in Claremorris, to raffles, draws, concerts, Christmas collections, coffee mornings, dances, fashion shows, sponsored swims, and bring and buy sales. In February 1985 the Board was told that £1.16 million had been collected in this way, of which the bulk had gone into the extension for the Linac costing £483,000 and the simulator and the simulator room which cost £246,000. The Friends have since gone from strength to strength, contributing over the 25 years as much as €22 million to the development of the hospital. (A full list of the purchases sponsored by the Friends is given in Appendix 4.) This represents a remarkable one-third of the hospital's total capital expenditure over the years since the Friends were founded.

### The cervical smear service

Another important activity that had logically established itself on the St Luke's campus was the National Cervical Cytology Screening service (cervical cancer had been the subject of one of Oliver Chance's first publications). The absolute number of Irish women dying from uterine cancer in the 1980s was 70 or fewer a year, a rate markedly lower than northern European countries and akin to Italy, Portugal, Spain and Greece, countries with similar traditions of sexual morality and stable marriages. [7] Nonetheless, the so-called 'Pap' cervical smear test had made it possible in this cancer to identify the cancerous lesions before the invasive stage. If caught early in this way, uterine cancer is almost 100 per cent curable.

During 1980–85 the centre examined some 40,000 smears a year, about a quarter of the national whole. Forty per cent of smears originated in the Dublin area. Such was the demand that the service was constantly falling behind. In April 1981 the Board was told that a backlog of tests had reached 15,000. An emergency injection of cash enabled the laboratory to catch up, but the problem, which was of course tied in with the general cash crisis during these years, arose again in 1983 when the Department made a special grant of £17,500 to clear a 7,000 item backlog; in 1985 the backlog had risen again to 14,000 and the Department granted £45,000; in April 1986 the Board was told that a new backlog of 6,000 smears had accumulated; this rose to 17,500 by December, implying a delay of 18 weeks, and the Department made another special grant, of £41,000.

Part of the problem was the fact that cytological examination is not an exact science. It took more than a year to train a laboratory technician to detect cancer cells under the microscope. The inventor of the Pap test, George Papanocolaou himself, famously used to say that he could no more explain how he recognised a smear as positive than he could explain how to recognise a friend by describing his face.

In her study of the service Dr Áine Gallagher reported that about 88 per cent of smears were reported as negative, and 0.3 per cent as positive.[8] Between these were samples diagnosed as 'atypical' etc., and those whose specimen was indecipherable. It was St Luke's time-consuming policy to re-sample any apparent positives, and normal practice required that a consultant cyto-pathologist examine and report on such smears. Unfortunately, the hospital could afford only a part-time consultant cyto-pathologist and this, combined with a clumsy record-keeping system, undoubtedly led to delays in the service.

Dr Gallagher said that, 'due to cutbacks in staffing levels', the cytology service had been forced to suspend its service temporarily from 8 June 1987 to 1 December 1987 in order to complete the backlog of cervical smears prior to accepting further smears for cytology screening. During this time laboratories in the private sector analysed smears and when the service re-opened only a percentage of their original clients returned. In fact, the number of smears sent into St Luke's was halved, and there was no more talk of backlogs. Indeed, when Dr Gallagher's findings were raised in the Dáil in October 1991 the Minister was able to state that the cytology department was now processing smears within 24 hours.[9]

*In the wards*

The *Annual Report* of 1986 records that the hospital, which behind the scenes was struggling financially, seemed full of activity, though comparison with the 1980 report suggests that activity was slightly lower than it had been six years before. In light of the continuing upward trend of cancer incidence this was a matter for concern. There were just over 16,300 patient attendances that year, compared with 17,240 in 1980. They came from all over the country (with three from Northern Ireland). The bulk of these were seen in Dublin, but over 10,000 patients attended 13 peripheral clinics from Donegal to Waterford. Most patients received radiotherapy, from one of the five powerful machines—two cobalt machines, two 300 kV x-rays and the Linac.

The hospital's first Linac had originally been installed in October 1984 but had not been available for use on patients while a dispute with the radiographers was unsettled. This serious and intractable problem arose because in order to see as many patients as possible, despite regular break-downs of the aging machinery, the hospital paid regular overtime. The rates were based on those paid to the majority of radiographers in Ireland who worked on diagnostic x-rays machines and who, when 'on-call', could be summoned back into hospital at any time. Although conditions in St Luke's were considerably different, the radiographers were paid at these levels. By the time an Oireachtas committee noticed what was happening, the amounts being paid effectively doubled their salaries. It was expected that the new machine would eliminate the need for much of this overtime. As a result the income on which they relied, for example for mortgages, would cease. When the machine was installed the radiographers put themselves in the ethically uncomfortable position of refusing the best available treatment to patients.[10]

Between them these machines delivered 8,400 working hours in the year (in 1980 the figure had been 7,580). Some 800 surgical procedures were recorded in the operating theatre, half of which were plastic surgery of some sort. There were also nearly 4,000 diagnostic x-ray explorations, and 1500 nuclear medicine investigations.

But of course the hospital was not a factory, to be measured by how many hours the machines were in operation. Every night there were over 120 patients in the wards, often, as a patient survey at this time discovered, insomniac—perhaps in pain, perhaps dreading the treatments to come and anxious about the final outcome. However supportive the family, friendly the nurses and caring the doctors, this was a lonely experience in an unfamiliar environment.

On average the patients stayed 13 days, not quite a fortnight. As their once-taken-for-granted bodies struggled to overcome the toxic effects of radiation, for many this was a time for profound and unfamiliar contemplation. For the large proportion who survive their cancer, this period of enforced reflection is life-changing, and the wooded tranquillity of St Luke's was particularly conducive to such readjustments.

As Nuala Higgins put it, after a mastectomy, 'Now, five years on I can say that life is richer after cancer. Worries and care take on a different dimension. Why get uptight? Why the hassle? Life is sweet. I could be dead. So now I really enjoy each day as it comes.'[11] Consultant Dr Des Carney confirmed that 'cancer patients never forget their diagnosis or treatment, no matter how many years go by. The experience gained gives added meaning to their lives, and many "survivors" will say that the best thing that ever happened to them was that they were challenged by cancer. It changes their lives forever.'[12] A major element of this is the severity of the treatment. For although doctors were now allowing themselves cautiously to talk of continuing remission (though hardly yet cure) for a growing proportion of patients, there was never any doubt that to eradicate the growth the patients' bodies would be severely stressed.

Olive Pickering, diagnosed with non-Hodgkins lymphoma, knew this. Her experience was no doubt common.[13] She first came into St Luke's in August 1979.

> It was a long day; I was exhausted and weary with pain. Eventually I reached the ward, and radiotherapy commenced that evening. The doctor explained to [her husband] that I had 'massive' glands and was very ill. My upper body was so swollen that when I looked in the mirror my head appeared like a pea sitting on a tree trunk. I asked the radiologists how long it would take for the treatment to take effect. After a moment's silence and a knowing look between them, they suggested that I might notice a reduction in the swelling by the end of the week. How could I wait that long? What if the treatment failed? The outlook was depressing and I was worried. But next morning as I felt my shoulders I was sure the swelling had reduced, ever so slightly. The doctor assured me that it had. How gracious God had been to me! My body was sensitive to the treatment and this was certainly the Lord answering the prayers of my family and friends. The radiotherapy continued for three-and-a-half weeks. My swollen glands reduced, but the side-effects of the treatment were severe. My throat became extremely sore; swallowing

was almost unbearable. My mouth was habitually dry; I couldn't eat; my stomach felt ill. I lost weight. Some of my hair fell out, and I got weaker and weaker by the day.

When the treatment was over, she went home, and gradually the side effects wore off.

The next stage was chemotherapy, also administered in St Luke's.

I went for my first chemotherapy session in St Luke's a few days later. Two nights in hospital and home again was what I expected. Unfortunately, the administration of the drug was unsuccessful and I had to stay in hospital for a full two weeks. After this chemotherapy was administered on a monthly basis. I attended St Luke's as an out-patient and stayed with my mum while I recovered from the initial side-effect—vomiting . . . while my body reacted well to the drugs, my energy was poor during these months of treatment and I had to rest to keep my blood count from going too low. I was vulnerable to all the winter ailments and was warned to keep out of crowds so as to avoid infection. When the course of chemotherapy was completed in June 1980, x-rays and tests showed that my chest and neck were clear of the disease.[14]

About this time Dr Anne (Nancy) Hilliard interviewed a sample of cancer patients in St Luke's and St Vincent's for a study of the needs of cancer patients and their relatives.[15] The study, the first of its kind in Ireland, provides a snapshot of the experience of the cancer patient at that time, a world very different from today.

The extraordinary importance of the moment of communication of the cancer diagnosis was not well understood, and a minority of doctors (not necessarily the most insensitive) handled the event badly. The St Luke's study confirmed a shying away from telling the hard truth on the part of some of the profession. Most patients perceived great sensitivity on the part of the consultant who had told them of the diagnosis; but nearly one in five 'felt that the consultant's attitude left something to be desired.' Many had been told by someone other than their consultant, often the GP but sometimes a family member.

Anna Farmar's study of the care of Irish children dying of cancer at this time noted how '[parents] expressed gratitude when the medical team had conveyed the information clearly and honestly, had appeared to care about the child and had supported them in their distress; they felt hurt when the diagnosis had been thrust on them in public places, without regard for the emotional effect of such news.' Quoting a UK study, the author described how 'parents vividly remembered, even years later, how they were informed and how doctors responded to their distress.'[16]

As many as a quarter of St Luke's patients claimed that they had never been specifically told of their diagnosis. Indeed about one patient in twenty either didn't want to know what was wrong with them or were unsure. Comparison with US data suggested that these proportions corresponded roughly to what was experienced there.

The still undeveloped state of palliative medicine was reflected in the physical symptoms the patients reported. Pain, insomnia and lassitude (weakness, exhaustion) were the three major symptoms experienced after diagnosis, although psychological problems such as anxiety, sexual dysfunction and depression were also common. Unsurprisingly, the study discovered that 'anxiety was greater among newly diagnosed and terminal patients than among the intermediate.' The clinical significance of this finding is not clear. A very ill patient, especially one expecting severe pain 'as a natural concomitant of their illness' as so many did, can perhaps be forgiven for feeling both anxious and depressed.

Although patients on the whole were satisfied with their care in hospital, pain control was then pitifully inadequate. Over half reported pain, and one-third of the terminally ill patients experienced unrelieved severe pain. Pain initiated a vicious circle causing increased anxiety, depressive feelings and insomnia which in turn reduced tolerance of pain. For many patients and their relatives this was no more than was to be expected. 'Most members of the public,' reported the study, 'think of severe and unremitting pain as a natural consequence of cancer and it may also be seen as an inevitable concomitant of cancer therapy.' The medical professions were not particularly well informed either. A US study of children's cancer pain noted that in the nine most commonly used paediatric medicine textbooks in North America there was a total of 3½ pages on pain management out of a total of 15,742.[17] Exaggerated fears of narcotic painkillers led patients into hiding symptoms even from their relatives.

These findings were more than echoed on the occasion of the launch of the Irish Hospice Foundation in April 1986. After a *Today Tonight* programme on RTÉ had highlighted the suffering which a scarcity of hospice and palliative care brought to people with terminal illness, the new foundation hosted a phone-in. Dr Antoin Murphy of Trinity College remembers story after story of relatives dying in agony. 'They were absolutely harrowing. It seemed there was a reluctance on the part of many medical practitioners to give opiates in the course of treatment. People were dying in the most acute pain.'[18] The modern cancer patient has to thank the hospice movement for enormous improvements in this area.

### St Luke's and St Anne's

It was generally believed in the 1980s that there would probably be some 10–12,000 new cancer cases a year, and that half of those would be suitable for treatment by radiotherapy. (These estimates are now far too low. The recent report by an expert group chaired by Professor Donal Hollywood recorded some 20,000 new cases every year, which was expected to rise with the population to 27,000 in 2015.[19]) A consultant radiotherapist was reckoned to be able to handle about 400 new cases a year, which meant 15 for the whole country. The question arose as to how these doctors and their expensive equipment would best be disposed.

Even then, the general policy of the Department was that individual specialties should be planned not as separate hospitals but as part of a general hospital campus. The serious problem of in-hospital infections such as MRSA had not yet arisen. Of course, the Department knew well that the existence in Dublin of thriving separate maternity, paediatric and cancer hospitals, not to mention straitened resources, made this policy more of an aspiration than a practical reality. Except, that was, in Cork, where St Agatha's Clinic had been folded into the new Cork Regional Hospital.

The problem of 'The future organisation of radiotherapy service in Ireland' (which in effect meant in Dublin), to take the name of a working group paper that first addressed the problem in 1983, overshadowed the board's activities between then and the eventual amalgamation of St Luke's and St Anne's in 1988. By the mid-1980s Hume Street had written itself out of the loop, having decided to concentrate on skin diseases.

After so long a rivalry, developing structures whereby the two hospitals could work together was a contentious process, filled with mutual suspicion. The Sisters of St Anne's, as the smaller hospital of the two, seemed to the St Luke's team both demanding and tenacious in attempting to ensure the survival of their institution. The consultants on both sides were unenthusiastic, and often uncooperative, fearing curtailment of their medical freedom. One meeting had to be wound up abruptly when a consultant on the St Anne's team simply lost his temper and began abusing the other side. As is usual in such discussions, the problem was conceived as a practical, operational one, and there was no call to consult patients' views.

Eventually, however, an agreement was reached and the 'St Luke's and St Anne's Board (Establishment) Order 1988', was signed by Minister O'Hanlon in December 1987. A new integrated Board was established and Reggie Redmond, in recognition of what the Minister referred to as his 'major contribution towards the integration of the services of the two hospitals', was made the first Chairman. The marriage, however, was made in the Department—not in heaven.

The years of discussion had certainly not reconciled the consultants. The new Selectron machine was a cause of contention, and when it eventually was located in St Anne's many believed that the Medical Director, Dr Michael O'Halloran, brought forward his retirement by several months in disapproval.[20] Whatever the truth of this story, it is certain that his effective successor, Dr Healy, retained severe reservations about the new arrangements.

This uneasy relationship was not, however, destined to last. In the mid-1980s the Daughters of Charity became interested in a new vocation in the burgeoning idea of hospice. With the help of the Irish Hospice Foundation and a significant donation from Michael Smurfit, St Francis Hospice in Raheny was established. The first step was taken in December 1988 when a Portacabin was cumbrously lowered into a yard next to the Capuchin friary in Raheny. A home care service was launched from this Portacabin the following September, and Sisters from St Anne's began to be allocated there. A new building with a day-care centre was opened in 1995 and a 19-bed in-patient unit in 1996. The Sisters' involvement in St Anne's was waning, and in July 1999 the assets and staff of the combined St Luke's and St Anne's hospital were formally transferred to St Luke's.[21]

By this time St Luke's itself had turned a significant corner. As the economy at first stabilised and then started to grow in the 1990s, the awkward, messy, make-do-and-mend era of the 1980s was to be put behind. Expenditure on the health service increased by 10 and 11 per cent per year in the early 1990s. Generated by a sense that cancer was no longer an inevitable death sentence, a new openness about the disease aided fund-raising and investment. TDs and senators, sensing the public mood, raised the disease and its treatment more and more often in the Oireachtas. A new Board, led by ex-Guinness MD Brian Slowey, evolved a plan for the future of the hospital called 'Vision 2000', which would transform the old St Luke's.

# Chapter 7: Reversing years of neglect

Services for cancer patients were very poorly supported for thirty years or more from the 1960s. St Luke's, as the only hospital in the country specialising in cancer, suffered notably from this neglect. No doubt the state, struggling to re-establish the economy, had many competing calls on its funds, but there were other, deeper reasons for this neglect.

It was, for instance, difficult for the political system to spend much money on a disease considered so ill-omened that people were reluctant even to say the word. An Irish politician of the 1970s or 1980s could hardly claim boisterous credit for crusading efforts against the disease whisperingly referred to as 'the big C'. Doctors, patients, family and friends colluded in this. Sufferers from HIV/AIDS and their supporters did not make the same mistake.

Gradually, however, these secretive ways were being abandoned. In the 1970s the word 'cancer' was used on only 193 occasions in the Oireachtas in the whole decade; then in the 1980s on 360 occasions; in the 1990s on 1,066 occasions and on 2,104 occasions from 2000 to 2007. The growing public ease with the idea of cancer—people increasingly prepared to say publicly that they had cancer, or that their relatives had it, and so on—was an essential precursor to investing money to cope with it.

Another reason why the national services for cancer were so neglected was the bias inside the Department of Health for concentrating their work on institutions and systems rather than specific diseases. The major exception to this, the successful campaign against tuberculosis, had been driven by two quite exceptional men, James Deeny and Noel Browne. Their energy had led to the building of numerous sanatoria. However, these became redundant only a few years after being built as a result of the introduction of combined streptomycin/PAS treatment in the early 1950s. Because of their characteristic spread-out design the buildings were very difficult to re-use, and were in subsequent decades a constant reminder of the shortness of their useful life. This awkward consequence seems to have turned the official mind away from the idea of 'disease champions'.

The Department's lack of enthusiasm for the wider aspirations of the Cancer Association was typical. The 'normal' attitude of the Department is revealed in ex-Secretary Brendan Hensey's much reprinted textbook *The health services of Ireland,* in which causes of modern mortality or morbidity are scarcely mentioned, and the whole focus is on the practical and legal questions of how hospitals and community services are organised and paid for.[1] Departmental insider Ruth Barrington's definitive description of the growth of the modern medical service has the same bias.[2]

In practice also, both Ministers and Departmental officials were preoccupied with the growing demands of the general hospital service. They had long demonstrated a pragmatic unwillingness to confront the fierce loyalties that established institutions could generate, as we have seen in the case of St Anne's and Hume Street. This passivity had a long history. As early as 1932 the unexpected bonanza generated by the Hospital Sweepstake had raised the possibility of planning 'a hospital system on modern lines for the whole country'. But the Secretary of the Department of Local Government and Public Health foresaw trouble, declaring that 'it does not appear feasible or desirable' for the state to accept any liability in connection with hospitals or to subvert the voluntary hospitals. The best that could be done was 'to consult the governing bodies' of such hospitals to avoid overlap in services.[3]

The lack of a concerted strategy for cancer services revealed itself in many ways. The number of consultants in both medical and radiation oncology was, at the end of the 1980s, less than one-third what international standards recommended. This meant that these specialists were having to look after as many as 800 new cases a year. Despite enormous strides in the field overseas, there were still only four medical oncologists in the country, all of whom were based in Dublin.[4] They were attempting to cope with some 20,000 new cancer cases a year. There was no national cancer registry to monitor incidence of the disease. Although breast cancer was known to be the leading cause of deaths of Irish women under sixty, basic screening was sketchy or non-existent; such mammography as existed was diagnostic. Cervical cancer could be discovered and cured as a result of screening, but take-up of the service was almost random, precariously depending on the energy and enthusiasm of local GPs, who could do nothing if they were not consulted. Cigarette smoking in offices and public spaces was normal. The Irish diet was notoriously heavy on fries and weak on fresh fruit and vegetables. As a result, Irish death rates from cancers of the breast, the lung, the colon and the rectum were well above European averages.[5]

A third element may perhaps be identified. Both medical (chemotherapy) and radiation oncology were becoming increasingly science-based and expensive. The drugs used for chemotherapy were enormously costly, and the early medical oncologists, such as Dr Fennelly and Dr Peter Daly (appointed to St James's in 1985), were conscious that scrutinising eyes were watching their successes and failures. 'To some extent,' said Peter Daly, 'we tried to choose the most hopeful cases to work with, so as to justify the techniques.'[6] There was plenty of choice. Sadly, the remarkable international advances of the 1960–85 period in leukaemias, lymphomas and testicular cancers were not supported by adequate consultant coverage.[7]

If the cost of chemotherapy was causing difficulties the same could also be said of investment in radiation equipment. Constant developments in radiation technology make it desirable for maximum curative effect that machines are replaced every ten years or so—in St Luke's the oldest machines were 25 years old. This was the medical equivalent of watching Sky Sports on a black and white television. It worked, up to a point, but at a cost. Not only did these old machines constantly break down, but they were not as flexible or precise as their successors—which for the patients meant that the lack of precise focusing greatly increased debilitating side-effects and sometimes tumours could not be addressed at all. In times of financial stringency, when beds were being closed and staff laid off, it is perhaps not surprising that the technically intimidating decision to invest in high-tech equipment was postponed. Consequently, new imaging techniques such as MRI were only available to patients in the Mater Private and other such establishments [8]

In the meantime, the Board of the newly combined hospitals met in January 1989, the membership consisting of five members from St Luke's and five from St Anne's. Neither John Healy, who had been 'Consultant in Administrative Charge' for a series of six-month appointments since 1989, nor Michael Moriarty, who succeeded him as 'Chairman of the Medical Staff Committee' in March 1992 and then as 'Chief of Radiotherapy and Oncology' some months later, was on the Board. This persistent exclusion of the consultants, which dated back to Oliver Chance's day, had long caused resentment.

For the first two years of the term of the Board Reggie Redmond was again Chairman, and then, following the finicky arrangement that betrayed the lack of true bonding, Kevin O'Donnell, on behalf of the St Anne's side, took over for the following two years. One of the old Board's last tasks had been to appoint a replacement to the Secretary-Manager Kathleen Rochford who retired in December 1987. In light of the new challenges, it was decided to upgrade the post, and in July Robert Martin joined the new organisation as Chief Executive. The hospital committee, that had been so involved in the day-to-day running, was disbanded.

Robert Martin's task was not enviable. St Luke's was still the premier radiation therapy site in the country, but its services had been run on a shoestring for years, and the new Chief Executive could have been forgiven for wondering about the long term. Key activity statistics such as bed days and attendances were far down on the 1980 figures,

Not only was the activity declining, but there were also teething problems with the amalgamation. Month after month the new board was told of problems between the two sites. In February 1989, for instance, it was noted that there was a shortage of beds in St Luke's, but 'transfer of patients to St Anne's was not working satisfactorily';

*Key Activity figures (data from 4th quarter)*

|                  | 1980   | 1985   | 1987  | 1990  |
|------------------|--------|--------|-------|-------|
| New attendances  | 691    | 692    | 544   | 531   |
| New admissions   | 272    | 188    | 120   | 51    |
| Bed days         | 11,375 | 10,888 | 7,150 | 7,569 |

this was later discovered to be because the St Anne's radiographers only worked on a part-time basis. In March the Board was told that payroll and other accountancy systems between the two sites were incompatible. In July the staff fears surfaced in an article in *The Irish Times* reporting speculation that St Luke's was to be closed. Reggie Redmond went on television to reject this, and the Minister issued an equally strong denial. It could not be denied, however, that the so-called 'Code of Understanding' between the two hospitals, which seemed to privilege St Anne's, was causing fears among the staff of St Luke's. Another piece of bad publicity surfaced at Christmas, with *The Irish Times* reporting that the hospital was to close for the Christmas holiday.

In March 1990 the Board was told that there was no way in which consultants could be compelled to work with the St Anne's Selectron, although Michael Moriarty found that it worked satisfactorily. At this meeting a no-doubt exasperated Sr Bernadette MacMahon went so far as to declare that 'the effort to integrate the two hospitals was a meaningless exercise', a comment primarily based on the attitude of people in St Anne's. Hopes that Minister Rory O'Hanlon might be encouraged to bang heads together were not improved by the result of his unofficial visit to both hospitals in June.

His visit to St Anne's went well, but that to St Luke's was a disaster, echoing MacEntee's visit forty years before. Despite three or four days' notice, the Minister walked through the Therapy Department on Wednesday 21 March at 10.45 am, and was surprised to discover that there were no radiographers at their work stations and no patients. The Minister was then escorted to the laboratory (where the cervical smears, in arrears as usual, were done)—and there were again no staff to be seen. On to a sleepy Out-Patients' Department, where there was very little evidence of activity. The Minister certainly did not come away with an impression of a bustling specialty facility, grappling actively with Ireland's second killer disease.

Bryan Alton met Minister O'Hanlon a few days after the visit, and told the Board 'that the message must be conveyed to the hospital staff that the Minister has expressed opinions that were extremely strong and that the case of St Luke's has not benefited by the shortcomings of the day.'[9] A flurry of letters from Robert Martin to the line managers produced various revealing rationalisations, typified by the superintendent radiographer's comment that 'Dr O'Hanlon arrived in the Dept. during the coffee time. I feel that if there had been more communication between Management and the Therapy Dept., or if indeed Management were interested in how the Therapy Dept. was run, the situation would never have happened.' The strength of this response was however somewhat weakened by her concluding remark: 'Since the time of Dr O'Hanlon's visit, the Radiographers have been reminded about their coffee time schedule.'[10] The radiographers were often at odds with the Board. Not only was there the long-running dispute about 'on call' rates, but in November 1989 Superintendent Radiographer Geraldine O'Connell had told the Board that she did not agree with altering treatment times to accommodate a planned Ministerial visit. It would, she declared, 'make life very difficult.' The Board minuted that in future detailed records should be kept of any meetings between the CEO and Ms O'Connell.[11]

At an informal meeting in April 1990 Dr Niall Tierney of the Department (also a Board member) told Reggie Redmond that the overspending could not be allowed to continue: 'the position was critical, and urgent and firm action was needed.' Ominously, Dr Tierney added that 'the Department was running out of patience'. In June Chairman Reggie Redmond attended the Department for a meeting which he had expected to be about budget matters, but to his surprise he was faced with the Minister and three senior civil servants, including Dr Tierney. The Minister made it clear that any question of increased funding would depend on the preparation of a proper development plan. Over the next two years various plans, medical, corporate, strategic, were drafted and discussed, and these in the event formed the foundation underpinning the later strategy Vision 2000—but on the surface little seemed to change.

Behind the scenes, however, something was being done. A Departmental Review Group, on which Dr Tierney sat, reported in 1992 that 'lack of adequate [numbers of] consultant staff, poor equipment and the isolation of St Luke's-St Anne's service from the hospitals sector [were] major drawbacks in the delivery of cancer treatment.' The report commented adversely on the lack of leadership 'particularly at consultant level' in the two hospitals.[12] In retrospect, this report may be taken as signalling a major shift in the Department's thinking about St Luke's, towards a far more pro-active approach.[13] At this time, too, Taoiseach Albert Reynolds' wife Kathleen was being treated for breast cancer by Dr Des Carney and the Taoiseach, not unnaturally, became particularly conscious of cancer services. As evidence of the government's new seriousness, Reynolds approached Brian Slowey, the vice-chairman of Guinness worldwide, and asked him to chair a new heavyweight Board of St Luke's to take office in December 1992. Slowey, approaching retirement, felt that now was a good time 'to put something back'.[14] He was also motivated in his approach to 'this horrible disease', as he called it, by the memory of the death of his mother from breast cancer at the relatively early age of fifty-eight.

A veteran of many firms, including Cantrell & Cochrane, Aer Lingus and Guinness, Slowey had evolved his own technique for appraising a business, 'walking the pitch by himself' as he called it. On his appointment he spent hours looking into every aspect of St Luke's, from the toilets near the wards to the offices and waiting rooms. He was not impressed. In fact, as he put it later: 'I was appalled, I was incensed, I was angry, I was very hurt by what I saw. The place was a dump; the equipment was archaic.' Talking to management and staff as part of this exploratory process did not change this initial strongly emotional reaction. 'Some of the consultants were committed and worked hard but too many of the outside consultants simply saw the patients as a source of earnings. The nursing staff were frankly demoralised . . . In the radiotherapy department not only was the equipment ancient but it wasn't being worked efficiently, which of course meant that patients were not being treated quickly enough. Catering was a mess and the place itself was awful'—symbolised for him by the fact that several of the hospital's windows were so rotten they had to be nailed shut.

It should be remembered, of course, that this was the reaction of an outsider used to the highest standards—in the state of the health service finance in Ireland, it is likely that more than one Dublin hospital had maintenance problems with windows. Furthermore, Brian Slowey's judgement about morale clashes with insiders' memories and the testimony of patients; for most staff St Luke's was a happy place to work, and patients consistently reported high satisfaction. However, in the light of the custom and practice glaringly revealed by Rory O'Hanlon's visit, it would be difficult to argue that the use of the ageing equipment was efficient.

The Arabs, it is said, have a proverb: 'May I never have to endure what I could get used to'. In St Luke's patients and staff had for many years been ground down by the consequences of lack of money. It required a complete outsider, with no experience of the hospital system, to come in and see clearly what patients and staff had got used to. Slowey's sense of outrage (still strong fifteen years later), combined with an empowering sense that if necessary he could expect a sympathetic ear from the Taoiseach, was to drive a complete re-envisaging of the hospital. Government had decided, at last, that something should be done about St Luke's. The door was swinging stiffly open, and Brian Slowey was put in place to give it a vigorous shove.

The strong new Board contained five very experienced men in particular—the 'five musketeers' as Slowey called them—who were to be intimately and time-consumingly involved with the re-invigoration of the hospital over the next two years. These were Padraic White, former Managing Director of IDA Ireland, Derry O'Donovan, a senior AIB manager, Donal O'Mahony, ex-Departmental Secretary-General and Dr John Cooney, a consultant psychiatrist. Of course, while restructuring proceeded, the daily activities of the hospital could not simply be abandoned, the relationship with St Anne's was still problematic, and the very negative financial position had to be addressed.

On the sidelines were the representatives of the Daughters of Charity, notably Sr Bernadette. As Brian Slowey put it, 'Sr Bernadette was in touch with me four or five times a week, keeping in constant touch with what her feelings and ideas were about the various matters we had discussed.' Clearly, the amalgamation of the two hospitals was a problem—especially since the nuns did not have much regard for St Luke's. However, 'once the nuns realised that I had a commitment—then they gave their approval to the merger and to the other developments.' In April it was confirmed that a strategic plan would be drawn up, to begin in July 1993 which would have as its objective the creation of a centre of excellence[15] on one site.

To put flesh on the aspiration a working group was set up under the chairmanship of Chief Executive Robert Martin. Their final report, *Vision 2000* (as it was ambitiously called), was published in June 1993, a mere six months after the new Board took office. The work had of course been greatly speeded up by being able to build on previous reports. *Vision 2000* started by confirming in sober terms Brian Slowey's reaction to the state of the hospital. Acknowledging how the original objective to make St Luke's Hospital the main cancer treatment centre in the country had been overtaken by events, the report confirmed that for years the hospital had been low on the Department's agenda. As a result money had been tight, though in fact there had been some development of plant, with the second Linac coming on stream in 1986, and the third in 1989. Thus when another Linac was installed in Cork in 1990 there were four in the country—some one-fifth of the number international standards would require to service the population. The lack of equipment meant that hundreds of patients every year from the west and midlands did not receive the palliative or curative radiation treatment they would have been given as a matter of course if they had lived in Dublin or Cork.[16]

For the hospital and the staff the real difficulty was in the day-to-day running of the ageing equipment—in 1990, for instance, the board was told that in the first quarter of the year the three Linacs had been out of order for a total of 83 hours, the two cobalt machines for 50 hours and the x-ray machines for 22 hours. Every hour meant delays in treating patients, so that sometimes treatments went on late at night, which in turn increased the overtime bills. The actual status of the equipment in the combined hospitals is graphically demonstrated in a table from *Vision 2000*. The regular repetition of the phrase 'obsolete—still in service' is striking, the more so since years before St Luke's had been proudly proclaimed as 'the Minister's hospital'.

*1992 Equipment Survey*

| Location | Equipment | Acquired | Status |
|---|---|---|---|
| St Luke's | TLD equipment | | Obsolete |
| St Luke's | Cobalt 1 | 1962 | Obsolete—out of service |
| St Luke's | Deep x-ray therapy 1 | 1965 | Obsolete—still in service |
| St Luke's | Cobalt 2 | 1966 | Obsolete—still in service |
| St Luke's | Contact x-ray therapy 1 | 1968 | Obsolete—still in service |
| St Luke's | Deep x-ray therapy 2 | 1971 | Obsolete—still in service |
| St Anne's | Contact x-ray therapy 2 | 1973 | Obsolete—still in service |
| St Luke's | Diagnostic x-ray | 1973 | Obsolete |
| St Anne's | Contact x-ray therapy 3 | 1977 | Obsolete—still in service |
| St Luke's | Dosimetry equipment | 1977 | Needs updating |
| St Luke's | 8 MV Linac | 1981 | Very troublesome |
| St Luke's | Simulator | 1982 | Obsolete—still in service |
| St Luke's | Treatment planner | 1983 | Slow and lacks 3-D |
| St Luke's | Ultrasound | 1983 | Limited capability |
| St Luke's | 4 MV Linac 1 | 1984 | In good condition |
| St Anne's | Cobalt 3 | 1986 | In good condition |
| St Anne's | Selectron | 1989 | In good condition |
| St Luke's | 4 MV Linac 2 | 1989 | In good condition |
| St Luke's | Micro-selection HDR | 1992 | In good condition |

*Source:* p 25 supporting chapters to *Vision 2000*

In addition, the process of integrating St Luke's and St Anne's had not been a success, and the hospital was now faced with a substantial financial deficit. The 1992 accounts showed that this had now accumulated to just short of £1 million or one-eighth of turnover. A further over-run of £395,000 was projected for 1993. Not only that but, as *Vision 2000* reiterated, continuing its hardhitting summary of the problems faced, the 'significant weaknesses in the current equipment' seriously reduced its ability to deliver patient services. Over £3.5 million would be required to put things right.

Support services (such as imaging, endoscopy and pathology) were equally problematic; the available equipment for such functions was bluntly described as 'out of date and seriously inefficient'. Of particular concern was the ultimatum from the Radiological Protection Institute of Ireland that threatened to close down the hospital if safety requirements were not complied with. For Board member Padraic White this was one of the most shocking aspects of the situation. Despite the growing demand from the consultants for more sophisticated laboratory services, St Luke's had fallen behind the major acute hospitals in this respect, and would require extra resources to bring it into line with current practice.

Not only was the diagnostic and therapeutic equipment falling behind the times, so were the facilities for patients. The old-fashioned 46-bed open wards were no longer acceptable, nor were the arrangements for out-patient treatment rooms, waiting or changing rooms. The size of the wards occasionally meant that male and female patients were in the same area, and unnecessarily exposed patients to extremely distressing scenes: 'Patients may die without privacy for themselves or their families, and mobile out-patients must share common waiting areas with stretcher cases'. There was little practical recognition that cancer is a profoundly life-changing event; social counselling and special services and guidance to help the patients and their families through this period, now commonplace, were underdeveloped. As a whole the hospital was 'inadequately addressing the overall needs of patients and their families', resulting in 'worry and discomfort to all those involved'.

As well as considering the patients' path, the working party looked at the way the hospital was run. It found that 'roles and responsibilities of the heads of function' were undefined and unclear; that fulltime consultant cover from oncologists and radiotherapists was inadequate; and that the range of specialties in place did not adequately reflect the needs of the hospital. Some of the part-time consultant posts were vacant, in other cases the contracted services were inadequate, unnecessary or not provided. 'Overall, these consultant inputs,' declared the working group, 'represent an historical and haphazard build-up of associations, mainly on a personal basis, over the years.'

The nursing situation was hardly better. In an attempt to keep up numbers in the face of employment vetoes from the Department, the Board in the 1980s had resorted to the establishment of temporary nursing posts and also to the use of agency nursing staff. Not only was this expensive, thus adding to the deficit, but the time devoted to induction and training was wasteful of resources. This was particularly frustrating as the role of nurses in respect of cancer patients was expanding. They were becoming more and more central in helping patients cope with physical and psychological distress, in educating them as to side-effects of treatment and at the same time interacting with a growing range of specialists in the hospital itself. Unfortunately, although the *Vision 2000* report tactfully did not mention it, the fact that the four ward sisters had all been in the hospital for many years greatly inhibited new ideas in that area.

For various reasons the hospital had evolved ways of working that were, as *Vision 2000* put it, 'difficult to manage, conflict oriented and probably inefficient.' Work customs that had evolved over years and hardened to restrictive practices were common. Matters were not helped by the fact that operating procedures were not written down, and were consequently difficult to assess or alter.

On the other hand, the hospital had some major assets. Despite its problems, St Luke's was the major radiation therapy centre in the country; it had the established reputation of the medical and nursing staff; it had the strong caring culture that had distinguished it from the start; and it had the excellent location, so important for the psychological recovery of patients. Tens of thousands of patients had valued this care, and their experience was reflected in the support of the Friends of St Luke's, who had proved themselves extraordinarily effective as fundraisers over the years.

What then was St Luke's to do? The new mission promoted by the Board called for the hospital to become 'a centre of excellence in radiation therapy and a leading hospital in cancer treatment, cancer research, education and prevention'. This was broken down into five sub-objectives, including participation in cancer research through the newly-founded St Luke's Institute of Cancer Research.

The aspiration to excellence was, of course, easier to articulate than achieve. The pivotal decision was to abandon the experiment of twin sites, which simply had not worked. At last St Anne's and St Luke's were to be combined as one hospital on one site—which but for clerical resistance and Departmental lack of will should have happened forty years before. Indeed, the nuns maintained a formal resistance. The Matron of St Anne's insisted on a reservation to the strategic plan disassociating herself from the 'serious consequences to both staff and resources' of any such amalgamation; and in September, just after the opening by the nuns of St Francis' day-care centre in Raheny, the board minutes record a concern by Sr Bernadette at a story in the *Irish Medical News* reporting the imminent closure of St Anne's.

Nonetheless, the amalgamation of the two facilities was crucial. Not only did the plan envisage a net saving in pay and non-pay elements of £490,000 following the transfer to St Luke's, but the equipment sited in St Anne's (including the Selectron, over which so much negotiating time had been spent in the 1980s) would be a welcome addition to broadening the hospital's resources.

At the same meeting management consultant Michael Jacob, who had been brought in to help juggle all these balls, was asked to provide a timetable for the implementation of the plan. From this time until his contract came to an end in 1996 he was to prove a significant asset in the difficult process ahead. The Board minutes regularly record 'report from Michael Jacob'; for instance, in January 1994 on 'upgrading facilities in St Luke's and the refurbishment of the old nurses' home'; and in July 1994 'Michael Jacob reports on building costs—Department have offered £6m but this is not adequate, we need £7.8m'. In practice, however, the Minister and the Department had been convinced by the case put by Brian Slowey (managed with adroit advice provided by Donal O'Mahony on the rituals of relating to senior civil servants). The proposals had, after all, been prefigured by the Tierney report and others, and they were no doubt very happy to see someone who was determined to make things

happen. In December 1993 Minister Brendan Howlin formally confirmed his agreement with the strategic plan in the Dáil.[17] Specifically,
he endorsed 'the transfer of acute services from St Anne's to the St
Luke's Hospital campus', which represented the opportunity for 'a
significant advance in the whole area of cancer care.'

Not that the plan was by any means out of the woods. In February
1994 it was realised that the finance allocation would give a shortfall
of £947,000 which obviously had, as the minutes put it, 'serious
implications for the strategic plan'. A good part of this shortfall was
generated by the radiographers' 'on-call' overtime rates which were
feared might amount to £750,000 that year. Given the sensitivities
of the position, successive Ministers had proved extremely reluctant
to address the anomaly that the radiographers were paid unit rates
based on genuine call-outs rather than the more appropriate time-
based overtime.

Gradually the new Board took the opportunity of retirements to
build up a newly sophisticated senior staff cadre. In September 1993
Drs John Armstrong and Donal Hollywood (successive Medical
Directors) were appointed; in April 1995 Eileen Maher came from
the Blackrock Clinic to be the new Director of Nursing; and in
December Brendan McClean, following the early retirement of Chief
Physicist Paddy Coughlan, came from Canada to take that post.

The recruitment process for the senior post of Chief Physicist
tellingly revealed how far the hospital had abandoned the international focus that had led the very first staff advertisements to require
foreign language skills. Initially, Brendan McClean had even been
expected to pay his own fare to Dublin; only after well-placed internal pressure from Michael Moriarty did a call come (at 3 am
Canadian time—the hospital had forgotten about international time
zones) saying they would pay.[18] He then got a brisk two-line letter
requesting his attendance at 8 am, but with no indication as to how
to get to the hospital or where he might stay overnight. When he
arrived he was immediately ushered into the board room where he
was faced, in civil service style, by a panel of 13 members (including
two specialists from the UK). He was not given any background
materials, nor asked, as he expected, to make a presentation; he was

not shown the equipment nor introduced to his potential colleagues. Only after the interview did Michael Jacob privately catch his arm, and say: 'Look, we like you—why not stay for a day or two and meet some people.' His hotel expenses were paid, and he met Michael Moriarty and others. Although amazed by the 'old and tired-looking' equipment, he could see that much was being done, and decided to join.

Starting work on Friday 13 December 1995, Brendan McClean was even more astonished, a few weeks later, to be summoned to the District Court as a witness. His brief was to explain how unlicensed radioactive sources had been found in a back room in St Anne's. So seriously did the hospital take this prosecution by the Radiological Protection Institute that Senior Counsel Adrian Hardiman (now on the Supreme Court) was engaged for the defence. Thorough investigation of St Anne's scattered and poorly documented holdings revealed that the Physics Department had been quite casual with the unwanted radioactive sources that had been deposited there, coming from Hume Street and many other places. One of the still dangerous sources, from a local doctor, had been given to St Anne's in a Mick McQuaid tobacco tin. As it happened, the District Justice did not progress the case, but no doubt the RPII felt they had made their point. A substantial and expensive clean-up of all the radioactive sources was put in hand. To Brendan McClean's eye, trained in the most advanced Canadian facilities, the storage methods in St Luke's, though fully licensed, were scarcely less casual.

In the meantime, in November 1994, after the surprisingly short tenure of two years had elapsed, the Slowey Board had been largely reappointed by Michael Noonan, the new Fine Gael Minister for Health in the rainbow government. However, since it was obviously impossible for someone of the wrong political persuasion to help in running a cancer hospital, two of the 'five musketeers', Padraic White and Derry O'Donovan, both closely associated with Fianna Fáil, were not reappointed. Albert Reynolds' close associate Michael Doherty was also not re-appointed. In their places came Frank Flannery of Rehab Ireland, Paddy Shanley and former Chairman

Kevin O'Donnell. Norma Smurfit did not take up her appointment. This board was initially to serve for two years, until November 1997, but its mandate was renewed until June 1998.

The reconfiguring of the hospital progressed in another area. In March 1996 Brian Slowey presented his radical ideas about a new 'Agreement of Understanding' with St Vincent's. This involved Robert Martin moving to a new job in St Vincent's while Nicky Jermyn, who was to remain CEO of St Vincent's, was also to become CEO of St Luke's. In his Chairman's memorandum to staff describing this move, Brian Slowey stressed the continuing autonomy of the two hospitals. Nonetheless, many commentators not unreasonably saw this as the first move in some kind of planned merger of the two hospitals. At the same time, the business of re-equipping the hospital also progressed. The ever-loyal and effective Friends of St Luke's had already agreed to fund the refurbishment of the nurses' home, now Oakland Lodge, and in July 1994 they had committed themselves to finding £800,000 towards the development project. With this and the sale of land valued at £1.9 million the Department declared itself in September 1996 prepared to sanction a third new Linac, a cobalt machine, a simulator and a contact therapy machine. A new buzz was being created in the hospital.

Two months later the first cancer strategy for Ireland for forty years was published by the Department.[19] Noting that cancer accounted for one-third of all deaths in the under-65s and that Ireland had a higher mortality from cancer than the EU average, it proposed a medium-term target to 'reduce the death rate from cancer in the under-65 age group by 15 per cent in the ten-year period from 1994'. In December 2003 the then Minister Micheál Martin was happy to announce that this perhaps too modest target had in fact been surpassed.

To achieve this over €500 million had been invested in cancer services; nearly ninety new consultants had been appointed; a national cancer registry had been set up; and multiple screening and prevention programmes had been established. At last the services for cancer were being given attention. There had in fact been a major switch from the long years of neglect after the slow strangling of the ambitious Cancer Association of Ireland, and the moment of the switch had been signalled by what was happening in St Luke's.

The evident failure, for human and practical reasons, of the proposed amalgamation of St Luke's and St Anne's, combined with the obvious consequences of so long a starving of funds for capital expenditure, had made it at last clear to the Department in the early 1990s that St Luke's was a 'suitable case for treatment'. The unfortunate Ministerial visit in March 1990 no doubt gave history a nudge, as did the chance that Albert Reynolds' wife was being treated for cancer. So when, as a result of the Taoiseach's intervention, Brian Slowey entered the scene with his vivid shock at the current conditions of the hospital combined with an enlarged feeling for what might be possible, radical change was in the air. The time was ripe, the personnel, including a powerful new Board, were in place, and finally the booming economy made the necessary investment eminently practical. As a result, what the National Cancer Strategy called in 1996 'the largest single investment in cancer services in recent years' was poured into St Luke's.[20] We shall see, in the last chapter of this history, what was made of this investment.

# Chapter 8: A haven still in Rathgar

In the 1990s it began to be possible to see cancer as not simply a death sentence. As Dr Harry Comber, Director of the Irish National Cancer Register, pointed out recently, 'nobody has yet found a cure for cancer' but the survival rates are inching up by 2 per cent every year. If this continues, he foresees that 'cancer will become a chronic rather than a terminal disease, a bit like HIV.'[1] Many cancers, if caught early enough, can be treated so as to provide the patient, if not with a cure, certainly with an improved life-chance. Perhaps the most spectacular change has been in acute lymphoblastic leukaemia which so often and so sadly strikes very young children. The long-term remission from this cancer is now above 90 per cent of cases. Similar success can be claimed for prostate, testicular and non-melanoma skin cancers.

This will enable cancer patients, as Blackrock Clinic radiologist Dr Doon O'Riordan put it, after her diagnosis, 'to live my life, not my death'.[2] Although initially unenthusiastic about the chemo-therapy regime suitable for her stage III ovarian cancer, Dr O'Riordan was persuaded by colleagues. A maintenance regime of chemotherapy once a week gave her a few more years of life, which included the opportunity to fulfil lifetime ambitions such as travelling to Canada and New Zealand, snorkelling on the Great Barrier Reef and seeing the Northern Lights.

*A very frightening experience*

Nonetheless, the increasing number of cancer narratives demon-strates that the cancer experience remains frightening and profoundly life-changing. For some the psychological shock is devastating. Gloria Hunniford's daughter Caron was not alone in being tormented with

the idea that her breast cancer arose because she had done something that turned God against her— 'she explored this over and
over again with different people, gurus, healers, spiritual leaders for
almost the rest of her life'.[3]

In her angry and emotional book *If it were just cancer* Janette
Byrne vividly catalogues the pains and indignities she went through
in the Mater after her non-Hodgkins lymphoma was finally diagnosed. [4] (As it happens, she did not have radiotherapy, but no doubt
many of St Luke's patients had similar experiences.) In her high-
octane style she describes the initial diagnosis (after some months
of going to her GP with recurrent symptoms). In the hospital they
found an advanced tumour in her throat, about the size of a cigarette
packet—'now the scans show a tumour staring back at us . . .
growing, crawling, choking, attaching itself to my windpipe.'

A strong theme in her account is how the practices and routines
in the crowded acute hospital barely acknowledge her as a person.
First the routines of the skimpy green gown affront her modesty;
then surgery and awaking, with a tube down her throat, in intensive
care—'drips, machines, tubes, stitches and the long wait'—had to
be endured. After three days she was moved to another ward for
chemotherapy. Here 'doctors arrive, white coats flapping . . . beds
are made, patients propped and cleaned, fresh air blowing through
the ward with no regard to its occupants. And we return to our duty
as sick people with a possible death sentence hanging over our heads,
waiting for it to tip one of us ever so lightly, letting us know we are
the chosen one.'

> These activities, along with the arrival of Dracula (as we humorously
> called the haematologist) begin each day. Dracula fills her little vials
> with our blood . . . we have become familiar with the blood levels
> needed to allow us home for a break. Most of us sleep poorly . . .
> because the chemo seems to heighten our sense of smell, the odour
> [of food] is enough to turn even the strongest stomach, [later] those
> of us well enough now stroll to the shop while others sneak out for a
> quick fag before the doctor's rounds . . . on those days when the
> consultants visit the wards I always sense the nervousness in the air.

Although the practical conditions are not the best in the small
ward, a strong and moving camaraderie builds up. 'Without the

girls I would have curled into a cocoon and I would not have had the chance to air lots of questions and doubts and would not have met the most wonderfully strong people who changed me forever . . . on the rare occasions when I saw tears—brought on by a poor scan result or a long painful day for one of us—we all seemed united in the suffering.'

Interestingly, it is the very shared experience of cancer that underpins this friendship. It is not the same

> . . . when someone is just in for a couple of days for something routine. Something happens on these days on the ward; it is as though a pause button is pressed on our feelings. There is less conversation and a crack forms in the support we give and get from each other . . . when it is just cancer patients on the ward there is an understanding, like a list of invisible rules in relation to noise . . . a genuine concern for each other prevails and an awareness of how tired, sick and strained someone can be from chemotherapy.

The novelist Lia Mills was diagnosed in May 2006 with cancer of the mouth. Her experiences in St James's and subsequently in St Luke's are vividly and movingly described in *In your face*.[5] Surgery involved removing a considerable part of her jaw and replacing it with titanium and grafts of skin and bone taken from her leg, at the same time cutting nerves in her face and tongue. She had a rough and painful time, struggling with the aftermath. A few weeks after the operation she is listed for radiotherapy, routine sessions enough, but vividly described by her writer's pen.

'St Luke's is small', she notes, 'and it never seems crowded as other hospitals do, although today is a busy day. It's a bright place, with fish tanks in the waiting areas, good art on the walls. People smile more here than I have noticed in other hospitals.' After a session with Professor Hollywood a mask is made of her shattered face. This is to enable exact targets for the radiation beam to be pinpointed and to make sure that when the radiation is occurring her face is immobile.

At another session, attempting to get the pointing exactly right 'they fasten the mask over my face and neck anchoring me to the table. They talk over me, numbers and angles and anatomical markers

. . . the machine moves with a lot of clicking and whirring; the table shifts up and down.'

Finally the real thing.

> They move the table from side to side, murmuring directions to each other as they position me so that radiation will be delivered to the precise area of my treatment field. They remember to talk to me too . . . whirring, wheezing, clicking, stops. A drone. The radiation therapists leave the room, tell me they'll be back soon. A high warning beep accompanies their receding footsteps like a lorry reversing. There's a pause, then the deeper, fiercer warning of the exposure button. They come back in to set me up for the next dose, given at a different angle and from a different direction. I don't feel anything—it's like having an ordinary x-ray. The actual irradiation only takes seconds for each field, and for me there are four fields, four exposures. Each time they reposition the machine they tell me what they're doing and when they are about to leave. I'm out of there in ten minutes, wondering what all the fuss was about.

Lia Mills has multiple sessions, so it becomes a familiar routine: 'While I'm enclosed in the shell I listen to the sounds of the equipment as it moves around me. I can track the buzz I hear back to the switch and on to the control panel, sending the radiation into action. I hear a high-pitched whine and imagine lethal darts unleashed on a search-and-destroy mission amid a swarm of metallic killer bees.' After the radiation there is usually a session with the soft-voiced physiotherapist, or perhaps a visit to the nurses' unit to check on her tubes.

### The mysteries of the cell

Very slowly biologists are unravelling the mysteries of the human cell, where cancers have their being. As we have seen, as late as the 1970s human cancer remained a black box. Since that time explorations into the stunning complexity of activity inside the human cell have confirmed that cancer is a disease of its deep inner workings.[6] The fault, it appears, starts in the genes, the great recipe book from which human life is created.

In addition, specific classes of genes have been identified as key culprits. The first type is comprised of 'onco-genes' and 'tumour suppressor' genes. They are respectively the accelerators and brakes of normal cell growth. Under healthy conditions they are programmed to control just the right amount of cell growth. In tumours, it is as if mutations have pinned the accelerator to the floor and prevented the brakes from working. The result is uncontrolled growth even when the cells' environment is persistently signalling for growth to stop.

One important discovery was the tumour-suppressing genes whose normal function is to shut down abnormal cells and inhibit growth. If these genes are defective, then defects caused by mutations in other genes are, as it were, 'let away with it'. As many as half of all cancers have been found to have defects in one of these, called TP53. Two others, BRCA1 and BRCA2, are important in breast cancer. Work by Dr Peter Daly of St James's and St Luke's in the early 1990s on an Irish family in which five out of six daughters had breast cancer was critical to the identification of BRCA2. Irish families of those days, being often quite large, provided an excellent testing ground for genetic research.

The second type are called 'caretaker' genes. These are the natural quality control inspectors whose normal role is to prevent defective or mutated genes from carrying out their function. Naturally, if a mutation renders the QC function inoperative, the chemical factory of the cell is uncontrolled.

There are dozens of different onco-genes and tumour suppressor genes expressing themselves through different chemical pathways in every cell. This means that there are always multiple ways in which they can go wrong. Traditionally, cancers have been described by the site in which they arise (breast, mouth, skin, stomach etc.); now scientists are beginning to be able to identify each specific cancer not by site, which is more or less irrelevant, but by the sequence of mutations in specific genes. The practical use of this was revealed with the new drug STI-571, which attacks the specific pathways that cause both chronic myelogenous leukaemia and the apparently unrelated stomach cancer GIST.

For a full-blown tumour with the ability to escape from the original location and invade distant sites, as many as six separate mutations may have to occur. The only difference between a benign and a malignant tumour is that the former has not acquired the last of these, the fatal ability to invade 'foreign' tissue. These so-called 'hallmarks of cancer' (see 'Six bad habits of cancer cells' below) show how complex cancer is. Lia Mills vividly experienced cancer as 'the crab, fizzing and spitting as with rage—that creepy feeling that it's trying to do its lethal work, embedding itself wherever it can find

## Six bad habits of cancer cells

| Normal cells | Cancer cells |
|---|---|
| Require external molecular signals as essential prompts before dividing | Deregulate normal growth signals thus allowing cells to grow regardless of external circumstance |
| Respond to specific anti-growth signals preventing cells from dividing until external circumstances are right | Shut off sensitivity to anti-growth signals |
| Are programmed to die in response to various internal and external signals | Have virtually all learned to evade the signals for cell death |
| Are limited in the number of times they can divide by a mechanism called telomere | Disable the telomere system so that they are able to go on dividing |
| Have a transitory and limited ability to grow new blood vessels in response, for instance, to injury | Acquire the ability to create new blood vessels independent of the rest of the body |
| Are tethered to their tissues of origin and are destroyed by the immune system if out of place | Are able to invade other tissues by changing the effects of cell-cell adhesion systems and cell-matrix links |

Source: based on D. Hanahan and R. Weinberg 'The hallmarks of cancer' *Cell* vol 100 7 January 2000 pp 57-70 purchase.'[7] In truth, however, cancer cells are not outside invaders, they are intimately part of the body.

## Continuing improvements

The reforms and renovations to St Luke's initiated by the *Vision 2000* plan were not incorporated in one fell swoop, but as a continuing series of developments. Extensions were built, and new equipment put in, with new staff to operate it. Donal O'Mahony, ex-Secretary-General of the Department of Transport, and Michael Jacob ran a subcommittee of the Board responsible for driving the process and minimising disturbance to the ongoing functions. All this involved considerable adjustments to normal working patterns, but the staff were delighted to see things happening and, as one insider put it, 'even the patients' happily put up with disruption for the sake of improvements. One simple but striking innovation was the placing of bright new works of art around the walls; this ongoing activity has been led by John Cooney, an art collector himself.

## A new constitution

By 1998 the hospital had been transformed. St Anne's had finally closed in December 1997 and the equipment and staff had at last moved to Rathgar. There were, of course, teething problems with the process of integration: every hospital, like every family, has a different way of doing the most basic things, as well as different styles, habits and customs which take a good deal of getting used to; for a long time nurses and other staff who had come from St Anne's were ever so slightly alien (in-laws, as you might say, rather than full family).

The term of office of the final Slowey Board came to an end in June 1998. And now there was an awkward hiatus. Nicky Jermyn and his team were obliged to continue running the hospital without a board for a full 18 months, while the Department was preparing a new Statutory Instrument governing the hospital. Although it was certainly awkward for senior management, it does not appear that the hospital's staff drew any bad conclusions from this lacuna. They were conscious that other places, for instance the Dental Hospital, had been without boards for various reasons.

To add to the confusion, in March 1999 Nicky Jermyn, who was already CEO of two hospitals, St Vincent's and St Luke's, was made temporary CEO of the new hospital in Tallaght. Outsiders must have been puzzled by the implication that there was only one administrator in the entire health service that the Department could trust.

At last, in December 1999, a new Board was appointed, under a new Statutory Instrument.[8] This document rewrote the constitution governing St Luke's following the folding-in of St Anne's. The Board's responsibility was identified specifically as the provision of a service 'for the diagnosis, treatment and care of cancer patients with particular emphasis on the provision of radiotherapy services'. St Luke's was to be 'a leading centre for cancer diagnosis, treatment, care, research, education and prevention . . . under the National Cancer Strategy.' The Board was to consist of ten members, appointed by the Minister though five were to be nominated by various bodies, for instance the Irish Cancer Society, the Irish College of General Practitioners, the Irish Hospice Foundation and St Vincent's. The Minister was also to nominate one of the ten to act as Chairperson. No remuneration other than expenses was to be paid to the members. Clause 20 (1) of the Statutory Instrument made it clear that there were going to be no problems such as the Cancer Association had raised: 'the Board shall submit estimates of income and expenditure . . . as may be required by the Minister, and shall furnish to the Minister any information' which he or she may require.

The Board, appointed by the Fianna Fáil Minister Brian Cowen, had as its chair Padraic White who, as we have seen, had already served two years with the first Slowey Board. Derry O'Donovan, another of the original 'five musketeers', came back to the Board at the same time. They had retained close contacts with Slowey and his colleagues, so were fully aware of the continuing process of development.

The new Board drew up a strategic plan which for the first time included specific financial controls to ensure that the hospital would at least break even, or even show a surplus every year. As a result of this business-like control St Luke's has not run a deficit for eight years.

One of the first tasks the Board had to address was the question of management. Although Nicky Jermyn was undoubtedly a good administrator, it was clear that if St Luke's was to progress it would need its own CEO. In December 2000, therefore, advertisements were placed seeking 'an experienced manager with a proven track record at senior management level in either the public or private sector, probably in healthcare.' The successful candidate, Lorcan Birthistle, took up the reins in April, moving from the Dental Hospital where he had been deputy chief executive. He had previously worked in the now closed Jervis Street and Richmond hospitals.

He had not been long in office when in October the *Sunday Tribune* reported that plans were being contemplated to close St Luke's. He strongly repudiated this suggestion, pointing out that in fact radiotherapy services needed to be increased substantially to meet international norms, and St Luke's was ideally placed to be the focus of such an increase. A development proposal which would have involved a further 80 beds (a 50 per cent increase) and four new Linacs was on the Minister's desk at the time. In September the Eastern Region Health Authority approved €2.9 million for the purchase of two new Linacs to replace those installed twenty years before.

### The future of St Luke's

Everyone was conscious that in May 2000 the Minister Micheál Martin had followed up on the 1996 National Cancer Strategy by appointing an Expert Working Group on radiation oncology services. The Group's task was to assess the future needs of Ireland's radiotherapy services and to advise how these needs might best be met. St Luke's future was obviously going to depend heavily on its conclusions. Appropriately, St Luke's staff were prominent. The group was chaired by Professor Donal Hollywood; John Armstrong, Brendan McClean and Eileen Maher were among the members. Board member Dr Sheelah Ryan, CEO of the Western Health Board, was also a member. The substantial presence of St Luke's staff on the Expert Group was in itself a recognition by the Department that the hospital and indeed the cancer problem itself had changed considerably.

The Expert Group's report was finally published in October 2003. It started by stressing the importance of radiotherapy in rather more than half of cancer cases. 'Failure to deliver modern radiation therapy', the report declared, 'can result in a reduced chance of patient cure.' There was no doubt that the national radiation service (exemplified by St Luke's) had been neglected for some thirty years between the early 1960s and the 1990s. Taking the simple measure of the number of Linacs, the basic work-horse radiation machine, in 2002 Ireland had 10 for a population approaching 4 million; Sweden had 56 Linacs for 9 million people, Norway 24 for 4.5 million and Denmark 27 for 5 million.

This was not merely through Departmental inadvertence. For years feelings recurred that radiation therapy was both crude and, with the rising use of chemotherapy, increasingly redundant. Articulate and passionate medical oncologists, led by forceful characters such as James Fennelly and John Crown, did little to correct this view. In 1995 Michael Moriarty told *Irish Medical News* how the Irish Society of Medical Oncology had proposed that radiotherapy and oncology be provided at major centres in the Mater and St Vincent's in Dublin and at centres on Cork and Galway. The logical conclusion of this plan would be closure of St Luke's (though after protest the Society subsequently reissued the report with fewer specifics about exactly where such centres should be located). Next, a group of radiation oncologists proposed that, on the contrary, there should be one major radiation centre in Dublin, based at St Luke's, and one each in Cork and Galway.[9] In an article in *Irish Medical News* in October 2000 John Crown called for 'larger, more muscular' institutions to care for cancer patients, bluntly declaring that the existence of St Luke's gave rise to a 'desperate mal-administration' of medical and nursing resources. Given this lack of professional consensus it is perhaps not surprising that the Department had been less than wholehearted in its support.

But the result was that patients, especially those outside Dublin, did not have anything like the radiotherapy service available that by international standards they should have. There were also puzzling regional variations in the use of radiation, and the time periods between diagnosis and commencement of therapy, that were not explained by the distance from a suitable centre. The Expert Group's prime objective was to plan how these neglected patients could quickly and effectively be brought into the net.

At the same time, important changes were being made in clinical radiation practice. Specifically, advanced computer-based imaging was enabling the radiologist to see the actual tumour in three dimensions and in real time, a major advance from the sophisticated guesswork that had gone before. Other developments included treatment regimes for certain cancers requiring pre-operative therapy; so-called 'hyper-fractionated' treatment plans providing treatment two or more times a day; use of radiation therapy in non-cancer conditions such as coronary artery and peripheral vascular disease; and deeper understanding of molecular genetics that was likely in ten or twenty years to enable radiotherapists to target critical pathways inside the tumour cells. It was Professor Hollywood's view that many of the discussions of the future of cancer services underestimated the potential future developments of radiation treatment.

These developments, as well as the inevitable increase in screening programmes, were going to require a considerably enhanced radiotherapy service. The question was: how should this be done? The answer was going to mean much for the future of St Luke's. The Group identified three potential models of service delivery, taken from international examples. The first was the development of a small number of big radiation oncology clinics, as part of what the jargon called 'multi-modality' facilities—the 'larger, more muscular' centres that John Crown had called for; the second was the establishment of numerous smaller centres across the country; the third was a mix of large and small centres, the so-called 'hub and spoke' model, which was an attempt to combine excellence with consideration of the patients' concerns about access.

But how important was this issue, really? Canadians and others were known to travel hundreds of miles to a centre of excellence. To explore how far access was a priority for patients, the Group sponsored a focus group survey. This put 'distance to travel to a clinic' as low as 13th in priority and 'providing the highest level of patient care' as number 1. This response seemed admirably clear, at least until critics claimed that the focus group was biased towards Dubliners, and (for obvious clinical reasons) the most sick were not included.

The focus group was also asked about current services. Although the experience in St Luke's was generally perceived very positively, the focus group was critical of some aspects of the care, such as machines breaking down causing delays, and most markedly multiple problems with communication including doctor to patient, hospital to GP and hospital to hospital. This communication problem had been identified ten years before in Anna Farmar's study of children with terminal cancer as being one of the most stressful aspects of such cases.[10] It was a major part of the argument for the large treatment centres that they would make the development and operation of close-knit multi-specialty teams much easier. In fact, as the science got more sophisticated, cancer care was anyway shifting from the days of 'my consultant' to 'my team'—as Lia Mills describes the 'max-fax' (maxilliary-facial) group that brought her through cancer of the mouth in St James's. Besides radiation therapists, oncologists and medical physicists, there should be quick access to specialist surgeons and medical oncologists, as well as to haematology, physiotherapy, dentistry, dietetics, genetics and psychological care.

Following this logic, the Expert Group proposed that in the immediate term, radiation services should be concentrated in large treatment centres, either based in an existing multi-speciality hospital or as part of a comprehensive cancer centre. Although the report did not say so, this resolved into a decision that there should be two major radiotherapy centres in Dublin, one in Cork and one in Galway.

The implications for St Luke's were obvious. To survive on its own it would have to persuade the Department to create what the

Cancer Association had always aimed for, a fully developed specialist cancer hospital with surgery (including substantial investment in intensive care units), chemotherapy and radiation. The three legs of the stool of cancer care, would, in this rather unlikely vision, be housed in the leafy seclusion of Rathgar.

Few doubted that the Hollywood Report's recommendations would produce the best technical medical environment. The argument about its conclusions arose because cancer is experienced not just as a disease but also as a profound psychological and physical disruption. In the Hollywood and Crown analyses such non-medical factors were not rated highly. Many patients and ex-patients, as well as the Friends, felt that to leave out the unquantifiable value of the special atmosphere of St Luke's was a mistake, and said so, loudly.

Following publication of the Report and its acceptance by the government, Mary Harney, the Minister for Health and Children, set up an international committee, chaired by her Chief Medical Officer Jim Kiely, to advise on the location of radiation oncology services in the Eastern region.

St Luke's was one of six Dublin hospitals invited to submit proposals.[11] It was in competition with St Vincent's, St James's and Tallaght hospitals to become the southside treatment centre. From the outset the odds were stacked against St Luke's, as the brief asked each proposer to argue that they should be the preferred location for radiation oncology as 'a component of a single-site integrated model' of cancer care. Undeterred, St Luke's now developed a detailed alternative proposal, with the help of international consultants McKinsey. Analysis of patient flows suggested that only a quarter of their patients would benefit from being on an acute hospital site, so the Board proposed a formal relationship with one or two acute hospitals on Dublin's southside. St Luke's would help them develop their radiotherapy expertise while facilitating its own patients to access their services. This was called the 'Single Service Multiple Site' model.

The international committee came to St Luke's in December 2004 to evaluate the proposal and the Board, management and medical staff presented their vision of St Luke's in the future. Then, as

Padraic White put it: 'anxious months followed as we awaited the outcome. By mid-May 2005 when Mary Harney came to St Luke's to open the extension to Oakland Lodge, there was still no news, but she assured us that she would consult us before any formal decision was announced.'

And she was as good as her word. On 22 July, she invited Padraic White and Lorcan Birthistle to meet her in her office in Hawkins House. Disappointingly, she told them that the international committee had come down in favour of St James's as the southside cancer care centre; on the other hand, she was committed to maintaining the expertise and ethos of St Luke's in the new arrangements which were to be put in place by 2011. As a practical demonstration of this she approved funding for the two new Linacs requested by the hospital and replacement of two others coming to the end of their life. She also asked her Special Advisor Oliver O'Connor to liaise with the hospital on the commitments to St Luke's to be part of the official announcement due shortly. These included the assurance that St Luke's would 'be central to the governance of the new facility' at St James's. In response to fears that the St Luke's site would be sold off, the Minister promised that the hospital would be involved in future discussions on the best use of the Rathgar complex.

To coincide with the official public announcement three days later of government approval of the national radiation oncology service, Padraic White called a special meeting of the Board. Having reviewed the outcome of the liaison with the Department, the Board and executive management issued a statement confirming their full support for 'the decisions announced today on the future development of radiotherapy services in Ireland and the East Coast in particular.' Senior officers of the Friends of St Luke's were specially briefed after the Board meeting that day and subsequently, after the initial shock, committed themselves to working on the new way forward with the hospital.

Although St Luke's had not won the coveted slot in the national radiotherapy network, the hospital was happy to take consolation from the fact that 2011 (subsequently extended to 2015) was some time away, and the Minister's announcement that the hospital would not be run down, but on the contrary new expansion would be encouraged. The decision was, nonetheless, depressing for staff morale. The Board took, and has sustained, a robust view. There were, after all, some 80,000 radiotherapy treatments to be delivered every year—nearly half a million before the then planned amalgamation date. So the programme of development and enhancement went on, if anything more vigorously. A special study of patient flows addressed delays in accessing radiotherapy services, and by a variety of measures average waiting times were cut, for instance for head and neck radiotherapy by 30 percent, and for cervical by nearly 50 per cent.[12] Extra attention was paid to landscaping the grounds and the development of rehabilitation services. In November 2005 chief executive Lorcan Birthistle announced a €7 million HSE-funded programme with the introduction of bunkers and radiotherapy space for two additional Linacs. And this was only the start of a continuing effort; in 2006 he told the Friends *Newsletter* of two replacement Linacs due in 2008 (in all representing a 25 per cent increase in capacity).

In December 2006 Padraic White announced that those four Linacs would be on stream in 2008. Smaller changes were continuous also. Car parking space was expanded, in conjunction with a considerable landscaping programme; in 2006, after a big push, (encouraged and invested in by the Board after a disappointing initial showing) St Luke's had come first in Ireland in the second Acute Hospital National Hygiene Audit. Following up a suggestion originally made by Dr Tim Gleeson, in spring 2004 the Out-Patients' Department was made available to a GP cooperative to provide a wekend and after-hours service for the locality. 'Lukedoc' as it is called, now sometimes has four or five doctors practising at once.

### A 'wonderful, homely, relaxed atmosphere'

But finally St Luke's is about the patients—and here it has a unique reputation. As a small, virtually single-function facility it is, of course, relatively easy to make life there pleasant. Emergencies and crises are less inclined to throw things out; queues are shorter; activities are on a human scale. To come to St Luke's for radiotherapy from an acute general hospital is like taking off in the crush and bustle of Dublin or Heathrow and landing in the relaxed calm of a small provincial airport. All patients coming to St Luke's have experienced their hectic times in a major hospital, so vividly described by Lia Mills and Janette Byrne. Now Janette Byrne, as the public face of Patients Together, often meets ex-patients from St Luke's who talk always of the 'wonderful, homely, relaxed atmosphere' there, in marked contrast to the Mater, in which she had found herself.

Of course, the praise for St Luke's is not achieved without care, effort and attention (nor is the praise universal, as complaints officer Marie Comiskey is aware). Patients really appreciate the fact that in a smaller, dedicated hospital they feel safe, the spaces and the flows are manageable, they can get to know the staff and above all everyone knows why they are there. A bit of mild competitiveness merely proves that everyone is still human—'someone mentions a woman who had fifty doses of radiotherapy, in tones that suggest that my twenty-eight are child's play', writes Lia Mills. And then there is a grey-faced woman in a wheelchair, bragging about all the different places her cancer has been found.

Dedicated facilities such as the Nursing Unit in radiotherapy or the Physiotherapy Department provide, as many report, a 'warm and supportive atmosphere'. As a comment on the web site RateMy Hospital put it: 'Given the nature of the illnesses of patients, the attitude, patience and professionalism has to be top class. And it certainly was from my perspective, from the catering staff up through nurses, interns and above.' 'St Luke's,' wrote another contributor, 'is a truly person-centred care facility that effectively maintains the dignity of each person and does everything in its power to promote the comfort of the people in its care. My father dreaded travelling to Dublin [from Leitrim] for his treatment but they provided an outstanding oasis of calm and comfort.'

It seems impossible that so much caring attention and so much goodwill should be lost.

# Notes

## Prologue

[1] Marie Harford from Rathmines, quoted in *Southside People* vol 11 no 15 11 April 2007

[2] For a detailed history of the house and grounds before the Cancer Association bought it in 1950, see Appendix 1.

[3] *The Irish Times* advertised the property as to be sold by public auction on 21 June 1950.

[4] The Irish Times *Irish Review and Annual* Dublin January 1951 p 57

[5] *Irish Architect* March/April 1991

[6] The opening is reported in *The Irish Times* 5 May 1954.

## Chapter 1

[1] M. Greaves *Cancer—the evolutionary legacy* Oxford 2000 pp 10–11

[2] See G. Lee *Leper hospitals in medieval Ireland* Dublin 1996 pp 46–50. The author suggests that Chapelizod is probably a corrupt version of Chapel Lazard, and that Leperstown was euphemistically changed to Leopardstown in the 19th century. Mercer's Hospital was built on the site of the leper hospital dedicated to St Stephen. St Stephen's Green is named after this foundation and the land formed part of the hospital's endowment.

[3] *Census of Ireland 1851 Part V Tables of Deaths* vol 1 Dublin 1856 part iii p 113. Sir William quotes the 1688 Bill of Mortality p 504.

[4] J. H, Bennett *Cancerous and cancroid growths* Edinburgh 1849 p 135

[5] See R. Buckman *Cancer is a word, not a sentence* London 2007 pp 11–15

[6] W. Whitla *Practice of medicine* London 1908 vol 1 p 156. Whitla was physician to the Royal Victoria Hospital, Belfast.

[7] Registrar General *Special Report on Cancer in Ireland* Cd 1450 Dublin 1903

[8] I am grateful to Sr Katherine Prendergast of the Daughters of Charity for copies of two documents describing the early days of St Anne's. Sr Louis Nicholson's *St Anne's Hospital* is primarily a memoir of Dr O'Brien; in 1976 a group of the Sisters compiled 'St Anne's down through the years' which carried the story to 1976 and includes extensive staff lists.

[9] C. O'Brien 'The cancer problem considered' *Studies* March 1924

[10] M. Lederman 'The early history of radiotherapy 1895–1939' *International Journal of Radiation Oncology* vol 7 Oxford 1981 p 640

[11] Although they very often, for instance on the cover of St Anne's *Annual Reports*, referred to themselves as 'Sisters of Charity' the more formal designation was 'Daughters of Charity of St Vincent de Paul'. Sr Louis Nicholson quotes a letter of 1927 from the Sister Provincial which begins 'The Sister of Charity . . .' and is signed 'Sister Mary Boyle, Provincial of the Daughters of Charity of St Vincent de Paul'. According to Fr Tom Davitt, archivist of the Vincentian Order in Ireland, the name was officially changed from Sisters to Daughters in July 1973.

[12] O'Brien 'The cancer problem considered' *Studies* March 1924

[13] Quoted in O'Brien 'The cancer problem considered'

[14] Registrar General *Annual Report 1928* Dublin 1929 p xxxii

[15] T. Mann *The magic mountain* Penguin edition Harmondsworth 1960 p 14

[16] W. Shakespeare 'Sonnet 35'

[17] 21 December 1922

[18] *Dail Debates* vol 64 19 November 1936

[19] I am grateful to Prof. Terence Dolan for this information. In the same spirit Tuberculosis was referred to in Irish as '*an cailín*'.

[20] I. Pearce *The gate of healing* Jersey 1983 p 138

[21] O. Chance 'Notes on the radiation treatment of cancer of the cervix' *Irish Journal of Medical Science* March 1941

[22] Registrar General *Annual Report 1936* p 52

[23] Registrar General *Annual Report 1936* p 50

[24] *Seanad Debates* vol 14, 1 July 1931

[25] M. Green et al *Growing up in Arcadia* Athlone 2003 p 2

[26] Note of a visit by Sir Edward Coey Bigger to members of the radium committee RDS 3 April 1933. I am grateful to Dr Fred Pfeiffer for letting me have sight of this and numerous other documents on the early history of radiography in Ireland that he has accumulated for his forthcoming biography of Dr Walter Stevenson.

[27] Department of Health A144/28

[28] The possessions of the moribund council are recorded (A144/28 p 57 and 58). They included a German dictionary and a copy of Cyril Scott's quackish *Victory over cancer without radium or surgery*; the meticulous listing of the contents of the office includes 3 wastepaper baskets, 2 ashtrays and '1 box rubber bands (half full)'.

[29] For the effects of the war on the Sweep, see T. Farmar *A history of Craig, Gardner & Co—the first 100 years* Dublin 1988 chap. 7

## Chapter 2

[1] Actually, it seems likely that researchers as early as the 1850s had noted the phenomenon, but it was Wilhelm Roentgen who carefully worked out the science. M. Lederman 'The early history of radiotherapy 1895–1939' in *International Journal of Radiation Oncology* vol 7 p 639 Oxford 1981. D. Porter 'The new photography' reprinted from the *Ulster Medical Journal* in J. Carr (ed.) *A century of medical radiation in Ireland* Dublin 1995 seems inclined to belittle Roentgen's achievement, describing Roentgen as 'stumbling on' his momentous discovery 'by chance'.

[2] See J. Murray 'The early formative years in Irish radiology' in J. Carr (ed.) *A century of medical radiation in Ireland* Dublin 1995

[3] See C. Norman Coleman 'Of what use is molecular biology to the practising radiation oncologist?' *Radiation and Oncology* 46 1998 117–125

[4] R. Mould *A century of x-rays and radioactivity in medicine* Bristol 1993 p 108

[5] Private communication from Dr John A. Murphy who worked in St Luke's in the 1960s

[6] R. A. Q. O'Meara 'The first four years' in *Irish Journal of Medical Science* no 349 Sixth Series Jan. 1955 p 3

[7] See T. Farmar *Patients, potions and physicians* Dublin 2004 p 166 for a discussion of how, as early as 1932, the cumulative and uncoordinated demands from over sixty hospitals amounted to three or four times what was historically an enormous sum. In self-defence the government had to establish the Hospitals Commission which in turn led to central authorities setting standards and generally coordinating hospital activity.

[8] *Quadragesimo Anno* Rome 1931 paragraph 79. Subsidiarity is undoubtedly a useful politico-social rule of thumb; it was an error to treat it as a moral issue.

[9] J. Watson *The double helix* New York 1968 p 18

[10] *The Irish Times* 20 February 1943. It is perhaps not surprising that the no-doubt classically-educated reporter was not comfortable with Schrodinger's exposition of the importance of negative entropy (where, as he helpfully explained, entropy = k logD), or his conclusion that the gene must be an aperiodic crystal structure.

[11] J. Deeny *To cure and to care* Dublin 1989 p 167

[12] Published in *Journal of the Medical Association of Éire* September 1947

[13] Department of Health 'Cancer' 23/5/1947 A144/28 pp 52–6

[14] *Irish Press* 23 April 1948

[15] Consultative Cancer Council *Report* Department of Health A144/9 pp 8–29

[16] S. Russ 'Historical background of radiation in cancer' in R. Raven (ed.) *Cancer* vol 5 London 1959

[17] Two members of the committee, Professors Victor Synge of Baggot Street

and R. A. Q. O'Meara of Trinity, showed how the mind of the majority was working by explicitly and formally rejecting the idea that the proposed Central Cancer Board should have 'coercive powers' over existing cancer hospitals.

[18] Department of Health A144/9 p 45, 46

[19] In a letter to Browne's successor, Russell refers to 'assurances which I was given at the time of my appointment by the previous Minister for Health Dr Noel Browne' (19 March 1953).

[20] Board minutes and a report of August 1951 from the Cancer Association to the Department (File M. 19 Minister for Health) detailing its activities: both in the St Luke's archive.

[21] I am grateful to David Murnaghan for unearthing and summarising this letter of 10 March 1950 from the McQuaid archive, and for sight of his MS 'Notes on Archbishop John Charles McQuaid and the Foundation of Saint Luke's Hospital'.

[22] Personal communication from Dr Finbarr Cross to David Murnaghan

[23] Letter from Archbishop McQuaid to Archbishop Dalton 8 September 1952 (sourced by David Murnaghan)

[24] Appendix 1, by Reggie Redmond, gives full details of the house and its history.

[25] Department of Health A/144.43 E70 et seq. January 1955

[26] Daughters of Charity 'St Anne's down through the years' unpublished typescript c 1976 p 23. I am grateful to Sr Katherine Prendergast for a copy of this document.

[27] Secretary of the Department of Health to Liam Egan 16 October 1951 File M. 19 Minister for Health

[28] Russell to Dr Seamus O'Riain 19 March 1953

[29] *Irish Architect* March/April 1991

## Chapter 3

[1] St Luke's archive 'Minister for Health file M19'

[2] Abbreviations: p. op. = post operative; CCU or CBU = carcinoma of cervical uterus, carcinoma of body of uterus; DXT = deep x-ray therapy; CXT = contact x-ray therapy; O.P. = out-patient.

[3] Guinea = £1 1 shilling issued as a coin 1663–1813 thereafter as a somewhat snobbish designation of price. Traditionally this was the unit charged by horse dealers and professionals, for instance Victorian barristers and medical consultants, with the odd shilling going to the clerk/porter/doorman.

[4] Departmental memo from Dr Deeny and Mr Owen Hargadon to Minister Seán MacEntee summarising the relationship between the Department and the Cancer Association 1957. Unfortunately for history the record of the relationship between the Department and the Association

is somewhat one-sided, since most of the surviving letters and papers are from Departmental sources.

[5] Thus expressed, for instance in the Cancer Association's first report to the Minister for Health, covering the period 10 Nov 1949 to 31 July 1951

[6] J. McGahern *Memoir* London 2005 p 210

[7] The Irish Times *Irish Review and Annual 1957* Dublin 1 January 1958

[8] See for instance *Statistical Abstract* Dublin 1957 Pr 4107

[9] The most recent figures reveal that in 2005 26 per cent of the 28,823 deaths were from malignant neoplasms.

[10] *Journal of the Irish Medical Association* January 1958 p 10

[11] Roosevelt has traditionally been associated with polio, and did much to stimulate research and rehabilitation programmes for the victims, notably the March of the Dimes he promoted when President. However, it now appears that many features of his illness, for instance its late onset, are more consistent with a diagnosis of Guillan-Barré syndrome, the so-called French polio.

[12] C. Cockburn *I, Claud* London 1967 p 375

[13] P. Cockburn *The broken boy* pb London 2006 p 28

[14] P. Cockburn *The broken boy* p 25

[15] S. Freud *Totem and taboo* translated by James Strachey pb London 1960 p 22

[16] *Model Housekeeping* June 1954 'Our Medical Bureau' column. The advice is repeated in so many words in November 1955.

[17] P. R. Peacock 'Carcinogenesis' in R. Raven *Cancer* vol 1 London 1957 chap. 4 pp 32–75

[18] K. Kinzler and B. Vogelstein 'Introduction' in K. Kinzler and B. Vogelstein *The Genetic basis of human cancer* 2nd ed New York 2002 p 3

[19] J. Feehan *Tomorrow to be brave* Cork 1972 p 38

[20] The law was clear that this was entirely the doctor's decision. A Supreme Court case in 1954 dismissed an attempt to sue a doctor because he had left part of a needle in his patient's body, but decided not to tell her about it. The judge, Kingsmill-Moore, declared 'I cannot admit any abstract duty to tell patients what is the matter with them, or in particular to say that a needle has been left in their tissues'. See Daniels *v* Heskin [1954] IR 73.

[21] J.McGahern *Memoir* London 2005 p 112

[22] The model Irish hospitals have unconsciously adopted is called in business 'ecosystem marketing'; in this practice the company builds such an intense net of dependancies and relationships around its products that it cannot be dislodged even by products known to function much better. Numerous technically excellent computer programs have failed to dislodge often mediocre Microsoft equivalents for this reason (*New Scientist* 29 November 1997).

23 J. Deeny *To cure and to care* Dublin 1989 p 142; Deeny notes that Ministers were 'very conscious of the "pork-barrel" effect of a new hospital in the community on jobs, contracts and prestige'.

24 Deeny *To cure and to care* Dublin 1989 p 167

25 From a Departmental memo dated '15 Bealtaine 1957' to the Minister summarising the relations between the Department and the Cancer Association. The affectation of expressing the month (and only the month) in Irish is characteristic of the Department's correspondence.

26 Eoin O'Malley, surgeon of the Mater, presidential address to the Medical Society University College Dublin quoted in *The Journal of the Irish Medical Association* January 1958 p 6

27 E. O'Malley *The Journal of the Irish Medical Association* January 1958 p 6. In 1953 the American Medical Association astonished the Irish establishment by severely criticising the quality of Irish medical training.

28 Departmental memo from Dr Deeny and Mr Owen Hargadon to Minister Seán MacEntee.

29 J. Deeny 'Mortality from cancer in Éire 1936–1945' *Journal of the Medical Association of Eire* September 1947 and 'Cancer mortality in the Republic of Ireland: a changing pattern' *Irish Journal of Medical Science* sixth series no 389 May 1958

30 Cancer Association board minutes June 1954. I am grateful to Reggie Redmond for his help in abstracting these minutes.

31 Internal memo drafted by Dr James Deeny 1957

32 Ted Russell to Reggie Redmond 15 February 1993

33 J. Deeny *To cure and to care* Dublin 1989 p 229

34 John E. Fogarty, the US House of Representative member from Rhode Island (1940–1967) was a strong and successful advocate for the rights of individuals with disabilities and an important force in the National Cancer Institute's fundraising activities.

35 Letter from Sean MacEntee to Deputy Russell 29 May 1957

36 When Reggie Redmond was appointed to the Board in 1958 MacEntee, a personal friend, sent him an annotated copy of this long statement, making it clear that his target was the so-called 'guiding spirits' of the Association, namely Ted Russell and R. E. Whelan.

37 Minister for Health files, E6

38 Memorandum and Articles of Association of the Cancer Association of Ireland clause 3 (u)

39 Seán MacEntee, Minister for Health, to Reggie Redmond 12 May 1959 St Luke's archive

## Chapter 4

1 F. Spear and J. Loutt 'Biological effects of radiation' in Carling et al. (eds) *British practice in radiation* London 1955. The copy consulted has the

stamp of the Cancer Association of Ireland and the date 26 August 1955.

[2] B. Windeyer 'Methods of radiotherapy: x-rays' in Carling et al. (eds) *British practice in radiation* London 1955

[3] Dail Eireann vol 178 25 November 1959; this reply was in answer to a question from Ted Russell.

[4] Department to Secretary, Cancer Association, 9 July 1960. St Luke's archive 'Cobalt Unit' file A. The echo of *Parkinson's Law*, especially the scene where a committee spend two and a half minutes approving the plans of a nuclear reactor, and three quarters of an hour discussing a bicycle shed, is unmistakable.

[5] *Sunday Review* 22 January 1961, and follow-up articles on 29 January, 5 and 19 February. This short-lived newspaper, edited by John Healy, was a subsidiary of The Irish Times. It was closed in 1963.

[6] Dáil Éireann vol 196 26 June 1962

[7] *Irish Independent* 23 August 1972. The review noted that Oliver Chance, a grandson of William Martin Murphy, had been on the Board of Independent Newspapers since 1928, serving latterly as vice-chairman. Coincidentally, the Chance family had paid for Noel Browne's education in the English public school, Beaumont.

[8] O. Chance 'Five years experience of arc therapy' *British Journal of Radiology* 1958 June 31 (366) p 293

[9] J. Byrne *If it were just cancer—a battle for dignity and life* Dublin 2006

[10] J. Steinbeck *The grapes of wrath* New York 1939 chap. 18

[11] S. Sontage *Illness as metaphor* New York 1978

[12] F. MacAnna *Bald head* Dublin 1988 p 24

[13] Fiction is of course 'made up' and so in a sense untrue. However, in such a realistic novel McGahern certainly presents us with what he expected his contemporary audience to accept as accurate or at least possible. Contemporary fiction of this sort therefore has a documentary value comparable to contemporary memoir, and quite different from memories written or spoken many years after the event. In fact, according to McGahern's *Memoir,* his aunt Maggie spent time in St Luke's in the early 1960s.

[14] *The Bell* December 1954

[15] The next few paragraphs are based on J. Patterson *The dread disease: cancer and modern American culture* Harvard 1987 especially pp 247–53.

[16] The researcher Dr Wilhelm Heuper spent a lifetime researching the impact of industrial pollution on cancer. He ended up as Director of the Environmental Cancer Section of the US National Cancer Institute. His work was publicised by *Silent Spring,* the 1962 bestseller by Rachel Carson.

[17] This was a common Greek sentiment: the quotation is from the last lines of Sophocles' *Oedipus Rex.*

[18] It is sad to think of the unhappy home life of the dinosaur discovered

with a brain tumour. A recent study of 29,595 Swedish twins born between 1926 and 1958 found no association between two personality traits, neuroticism and extraversion, and any group of cancer. These were the specific personality traits most commonly thought to contribute to cancer risk. *Cancer* March 2005.

[19] F. MacAnna *Bald head* Dublin 1988 p 18. 'Reminded me' is interesting, as if the power of the mind over cancerous growth were an established fact.

[20] *Woman's Way* 13 November 1970

[21] F. MacAnna *Bald head* Dublin 1988 p 16

[22] I. Heron *When trees were green* London 1978 pp 109–119, 201, 222

## Chapter 5

[1] 'Letter from Austin Darragh, founder of the Irish Cancer Society' read to the 40th anniversary dinner of the Society in October 2003

[2] William Norton, former leader of the Labour Party, Dáil Éireann vol 205 23 Oct 1963

[3] Report of the directors for the year 1966

[4] The quoted sentences are from the randomly picked minutes of the meeting 25 April 1974.

[5] Interview with Josephine Fitzmaurice, Breda Carroll and Phil Sutton May 2007

[6] The hospital committee sat on 25 April (a Thursday); either the social committee were seeking retrospective permission or (more likely) the date of 24 April is a mistake.

[7] J. McGahern *The Pornographer* London 1979 p 176. The real purpose of his visit is the entertainment he later receives in the nurses' home which includes scenes which former Personnel Manager Josephine FitzMaurice described to me as 'not entirely male fantasy'.

[8] J. McGahern *The Pornographer* London 1979 p 223

[9] Unfortunately, Prof. O'Halloran was unable to meet me during the course of the research for this book.

[10] J. O'Connor and P. Coughlan *Bulletin of the Hospital Physicists' Association* November 1969

[11] Before Chernobyl (1986) the Windscale fire and the Three Mile Island incident were the worst accidents in nuclear plants.

[12] D. Murnaghan 'Development of x-ray protection' in J. Carr *A century of medical radiation in Ireland* Dublin 1995 p 152. I am grateful to David Murnaghan for a personal interview and for a copy of a booklet of 1975 describing the NRMS services. This is now in the hospital's archive.

[13] J. Byrne *If it were just cancer* Dublin 2006 p 24

[14] J. Feehan *Tomorrow to be brave* Cork 1972 p 2

[15] A. Solzenitsyn *Cancer Ward* Harmondsworth 1971 p 340; R. Picardie *Before I say goodbye* London 1998 p 16

[16] In Temple Street Children's Hospital in the early 1980s nurses were forbidden to leave textbooks and reference materials lying around the nurses station lest the parents of the young patients gain access to undigested technical information. The well-equipped research resource centre in St Luke's is not open to patients.

[17] *Irish Medical News* 6 February 2006

[18] R. O'Meara 'Cancer research at St Luke's Hospital' in *Irish Journal of Medical Science* eighth series vol 3 no 2 February 1970 p 59

[19] J. Goodfield *Cancer under siege* London 1975 p 108

## Chapter 6

[1] B. Herity et al. *Cancer: Ireland and the EC* Dublin 1991 p 31

[2] R. Doll and R. Peto *The causes of cancer* Oxford 1981. First published in the *Journal of the National Cancer Insitute* vol 66 June 1981

[3] B. Herity et al *Cancer: Ireland and the EC* Dublin 1991

[4] M-A Wren *Unhealthy state* Dublin 2003 p 65

[5] Department of Health *Acute Hospital Bed Capacity Review* Dublin 2002. Almost all this increase was in day-bed procedures; over the same period the number of out-patients treated rose from 1.5 million to 2 million a year.

[6] Reggie Redmond to Dr Michael Woods TD 27 Aug 1980

[7] This is based on 'Cervical screening: an evaluation of the National Cervical Cytology Screening service', a thesis submitted for membership of the Faculty of Community Medicine of the RCPI by Dr Aine Gallagher in March 1989.

[8] A. Gallagher 'Cervical screening' p 3

[9] Nuala Fennell asked the question of Minister O'Hanlon; *Dáil Debates* vol 411 31 Oct 1991. When Mary Harney had raised the matter in 1988 the Minister talked of a one-week turn round.

[10] *Dáil Debates* vol 364 25 Feb 1986

[11] N. Higgins 'Seize the day!' in J. Briscoe and R. Collins (eds) *Talking cancer* Dublin 1996 p 38

[12] J. Briscoe and R. Collins (eds) *Talking cancer* Dublin 1996 pp 149–59

[13] Olive Pickering was the wife of the Rector of Drumcree who controversially insisted on keeping his church open for the annual parade of the Portadown Orangemen during the so-called Drumcree stand-off which began in 1995. She died in 2006. *Belfast Telegraph* 27 June 2007

[14] O. Pickering 'Forward in faith' in J. Briscoe and R. Collins (eds) *Talking Cancer* Dublin 1996 p 33

[15] A. Hilliard 'A survey of the needs of cancer patients and their relatives'; thesis submitted for membership of the RCPI Faculty of Community Medicine October 1985. The 200 or so patients were from St Luke's and from St Vincent's Oncology Centre. A summary was later published as

B. Herity et al. 'A study of the needs of cancer patients and their relatives' *Irish Journal of Medical Science* June 1987 pp 172–181.

[16] A. Farmar *Children's last days* Dublin 1992 pp 20–21

[17] Quoted in A. Farmar *Children's last days* Dublin 1992 p 101

[18] Quoted in P. O'Morain *The Irish Hospice Foundation 1986–2006* Dublin 2006 p 9

[19] Department of Health *The development of radiation oncology services in Ireland* Dublin, Stationery Office PRN 203 nd [2003]

[20] Since Prof. O'Halloran was unable to see me, I report this merely as hearsay. It is, however, indicative of the strength of the feelings generated by this shotgun marriage.

[21] *Saint Luke's and Saint Anne's Hospital Board (Revocation) Order 1999* SI no 252 of 1999 signed in July by Minister Brian Cowan.

## *Chapter 7*

[1] 4th edition 1988. Dr Hensey had been involved in the setting-up of the Department in 1947 and was Secretary 1973–81. I worked with Dr Hensey on a previous edition of this book, and well remember the over-riding concern he had for his role as financial reporting officer for the Department to the Oireachtas.

[2] R. Barrington *Health, medicine and politics in Ireland 1900–1970* Dublin 1987. Neither heart disease nor cancer is mentioned in the index. Ruth Barrington joined the Department of Health in 1973. Her father Tom worked in the Custom House at the time of the establishment of the Department before going on to set up the Institute of Public Administration.

[3] Edward McCarron, quoted in Mary E. Daly 'State and Dublin hospitals in the 1930s' in E. Malcolm and G. Jones *Medicine, disease and the state in Ireland 1650–1940* Cork 1999 p 242

[4] 'Treatment for cancer patients' *Dáil debates* 25 April 1995

[5] Department of Health *Cancer services in Ireland: a national strategy* Dublin November 1996 p 10

[6] Interview with Dr Peter Daly July 2007

[7] See J.Fennelly 'Major developments in cancer care in 25 years' *Irish Medical Times* 10 January 1992

[8] MRI scanners were commercially available in the US from 1980, and the Mater Private's expensive but justified decision was strongly influenced by personal experience in the US. See T. Farmar *Mater Private 1986–2006* Dublin 2006 pp 54–55

[9] Board minutes 23 May 1990

[10] Geraldine O'Connell to Robert Martin 11 June 1990. St Luke's archive. At the bottom of this letter Robert Martin has written crisply 'We appoint senior people in Depts. to manage'—a comment which says as

much about his approach as Ms O'Connell's.

[11] Board minutes November 1989

[12] *Irish Medical News* June 1992

[13] Official attitudes had begun to change in the 1990s. Documents such as *Shaping a healthier future* (1994) and *Cancer services in Ireland: a national cancer strategy* published in 1996 were evidence of this more proactive approach to health promotion.

[14] Interview with Brian Slowey September 2007

[15] The word 'excellence' had come into business vocabulary with Tom Peters' astonishingly successful business guru book *In search of excellence* published in 1982.

[16] Department of Health and Children *The development of radiation oncology services in Ireland* Dublin 2003

[17] *Dáil Debates* vol 437 16 December 1993

[18] Interview with Dr Brendan McClean August 2007

[19] Department of Health and Children *Cancer services in Ireland: a national strategy* Dublin 1996

[20] Department of Health and Children *Cancer Services in Ireland: A national strategy* Dublin 1996 p 31

## *Chapter 8*

[1] *The Irish Times* 13 February 2007

[2] *The Irish Times* 12 May 2006

[3] G. Hunniford *Next to you: Caron's courage remembered by her mother* London 2005 p 223

[4] J. Byrne *If it were just cancer* Dublin 2006; the quotations in this and the following paragraphs come from pages 15, 56, 92, 101–2.

[5] L. Mills *In your face* Dublin 2007 pp 144, 192, 206, 207

[6] What follows is based on B. Vogelstein and K. Kinzler *The genetic basis of human cancer* New York 2002 chapter 1

[7] L. Mills *In your face* Dublin 2007 p 33

[8] SI no 253 of 1999

[9] *Irish Medical News* 17 July 1995

[10] A. Farmar *Children's last days* Dublin 1992 p 46

[11] These paragraphs are based on detailed briefing by Chairman Padraic White.

[12] This Board subcommittee was established following an audit of patients' waiting times by Dr Clare Faul, Chair of the Department of Radiation Oncology, and Dr David FitzPatrick.

# The early history of Oakland
## *Reggie Redmond*

*Rath Garth*

In the centuries preceding the Anglo-Norman invasion the Viking town of Dyflin consisted of little more than a fortified settlement on the hill now occupied by Christ Church Cathedral. With the arrival of the Anglo-Normans in 1169 and the capture of Dublin the slow but steady growth of the city began. King John of England ordered the building of Dublin Castle in 1204 and this was completed in 1230.

During the following two or three centuries Dublin remained, by our standards, a very tiny city surrounded by walls and gates. The areas which we know today as College Green, St Stephen's Green and beyond were rural, whilst Rathgar consisted of farmland, forest and a few pathways.

Outside the walls of Dublin to the east, near the site of Trinity College, stood the Abbey of St Mary de Hogges, a convent for Augustinian nuns established in 1146 by the King of Leinster, Diarmuid MacMurrough. This was located close to College Green, and the area was known as Hoggen Green or the Hogges (meaning mounds). The Abbey also owned '90 acres of land containing a manor house, a granary and farm buildings' together with 3 acres of woodlands, all located in an area known then as Rath Garth. This is an anglicized version of the Irish 'Rath Garbh' meaning 'the rough fort' or 'rough land', 'uncultivated land'. John Taylor's map 'Environs of Dublin 1816' shows an earthen ring fort situated between the present-day Neville Road and Villiers Road. In early writings the name was also written as Rath Garr, and finally Rathgar. The Abbey farm would have occupied the area around St Luke's Hospital and the present village of Rathgar.

## Rathgar Castle

For many hundreds of years this farmland continued to provide produce and income for the 'nunnery'. However, during the 16th century the dissolution of the Irish religious houses had been ordered by Henry VIII and in 1539 the lands in 'Rathgarr' being owned by the Abbey were granted to one Nicholas Segrave. In 1609 what is described as 'A house, 6 messuages and 120 acres in Rathgar, Co. Dublin' came into the possession of Alderman John Cusack, the Mayor of Dublin. (The title Lord Mayor only came into use during the 18th century).

John Cusack was an Alderman from 1604 until his death on 30 May, 1626. He was Mayor from 1608 to 1609 and subsequently City Treasurer. He is described as a Merchant who had important trade with England. He came from a long-settled and prominent family in Co. Meath. His mother was Maud Plunkett, while his wife, Margaret, was the widow of Alderman John Gough who, himself, had held the office of Mayor in 1576. Cusack's daughter, Barbara, had married Edward, the son of another Mayor, Alderman John Arthur. An ancestor, Thomas Cusack, had in 1409 been appointed

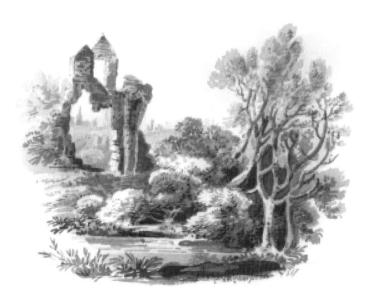

*A romantic image of the ruins of Rathgar Castle, with Dublin visible in the distance, by Cecilia Campbell (1816) (courtesy National Library)*

the first Mayor of Dublin. Thus John Cusack had, as we would say today, 'good connections'. He was a Protestant and is recorded as attending church services every Sunday during his mayoralty. In these years, in the wake of the Reformation, there was considerable tension on the City Council between the Catholic and Protestant aldermen.

Alderman Cusack was succeeded in Rathgar by his son Robert and eventually his grandson, Adam, and thus the family held the property as their residence for more than a century. There is no doubt that what eventually became known as Rathgar Castle was the original manor house described in early deeds. Its location is shown as 'Ruins' on John Taylor's map in the area of Fairfield Park.

In the 17th century Rathgar as a village did not exist and the area did not even straddle a main road out of Dublin. Rathgar Road is modern, being constructed around 1815. Highfield Road was just a farm track leading from Rathmines Castle, which was near the present-day site of Palmerston Park. (Temple Road is named after the family who had possession of that castle and lands in the early 18th century). Rathgar Avenue was an ancient avenue or pathway which gave access to Rathgar Castle from the Harold's Cross Road, which was the main road out of Dublin leading to Terenure and Rathfarnham. This avenue continued along the line of Orwell Road to the River Dodder where there was a ford at the site of Orwell Bridge (formerly Waldron's Bridge). It is probable that one of the main entrances to the Castle stood near Rathgar crossroads until very recently, as Weston St John Joyce wrote in 1912 'On Orwell Road, about 80 yards from the tram track, are the massive pillars of a gateway.'

The Battle of Rathmines, which is still part of the local folklore, took place in 1649. This was fought between the Royalists and the Parliamentarians (Cromwellians). Cromwell's forces, under Col. Michael Jones, had captured Baggotrath Castle, situated in the Pembroke Road/Baggot Street area, and as the defenders retreated Jones cut them off by marching his forces along the Dodder, past Donnybrook and then swinging around to face the Royalists at

Cullenswood in Ranelagh. The defeated army fled to the woods around Rathgar Castle and Jones has recorded, 'our men continued their pursuit and found a party of about two thousand foot in a grove belonging to Rathgar Castle, who after some defence, obtained conditions for their lives.' Rathmines Castle and Rathgar Castle, the Cusacks' residence, were both severely damaged at this time.

The castle was repaired and the Cusack family continued to live there for many more decades. However, eventually they started to lease portions of their lands to various dairymen and market gardeners. Legal deeds of those times indicate numerous leases by the Cusacks to various parties, including one Henry Coulson, after whose descendants Coulson Avenue was named. Another lease refers to '37 acres lands of Rathgar known as Sarah Ellis Farm'. An old title deed of 1757 records the sale by another John Cusack of a 'House' and the 'Mill of Rathgar' to one Redmond Morres, a non-resident landlord. Twelve years later Morres granted a lease to a Richard Wilson of '7 acres known as Clover Meadow on the upper end of new Cross Avenue (Highfield Road) on the left hand'. By this time the old Castle was in ruins, as can be seen in a painting done the same year (1769) by Gabriel Beranger, a Dutch Huguenot who lived in Ireland. In 1782 a well-known antiquarian Austin Cooper visited the area and as described in his 'Notebook' found only the walls and an entrance gateway still standing. This gateway is probably the 'massive pillars' which Joyce found in 1912, on Orwell Road. In a book of ballads, *The Monks of Kilcrea*, on page 121 is a story of Rathgar called 'The Rapparee's Tale' by an author named Geoghegan. The first verses are as follows:

> Rathgar, upon thy broken wall
> Now grows the lusmore* rank and tall–
> Wild grass upon thy hearthstone springs,
> And ivy round thy turret clings;
> The night owls through thy arches sweep,
> Thy moat dried up, thy towers aheap,
> Blackened and charr'd and desolate—
> The traveler marvels at thy fate!

But other look thy tall towers bore
Upon that well known night,
When silentlie we scaled the bawn
And stood beneath thy tall oak boughs,
Close sheltered from the sight
With bustle loud thy courtyards rung
As horsemen from their saddles sprung
All lightly to the ground.
*Lusmore—probably foxglove*

However, things were changing. The Wilsons had built a house which would become known as Rathgar House. A new and modern era was about to begin.

### Rathgar House

The house built for the Wilsons was described as being 'in the heart of the country' and was a much more modest structure than the 'Oakland' that we know today. Indeed it is not certain at all that the original house has survived. The pathway leading from Rathmines had been improved and was now a road (the Cross Avenue). An inn and some thatched cottages had been built at the crossroads (the area being called The Thatch) and thus Rathgar was opened up to travellers and trade.

The prospects were good. This road was by then called the Rathgar Road and, when the present day Rathgar Road was cut in a straight line up from Rathmines, it was called for a period, the Old Rathgar Road and finally in 1863 'Highfield Road'. Mr Wilson and family did not keep the property very long and about 1788 sold out to Charles Farran, a Freeman of the City of Dublin. The Farran name was to be associated with Rathgar House for three-quarters of a century.

Charles Farran was an attorney by profession and held the post of Clerk of the Pleas in the Court of the Exchequer. He was therefore a person of distinction and influence, and his presence in Rathgar must have accelerated the growth of the desolate crossroads into the nucleus of a village. Rathgar House was the first modern house to be build on Highfield Road, or indeed in Rathgar, and Farran was certainly in residence there prior to 16 May 1788, as his prayer book bears that date on the fly-leaf together with the inscription in his own handwriting 'This is the Property of Charles Farran of Rathgar in the Parish of Rathfarnham County Dublin.' His town residence was in Golden Lane, but by 1795 he is recorded as having moved to 50 York Street.

The next decade was that leading up to the Rising of 1798 and feelings were running high in all parts of the country. Mr Farran had an employee, Daniel Carroll, variously described as a gardener or a carter, who lived in a small gate-lodge on the estate. In the early hours of 16 March, 1798 an attack, which seems to have been partly politically motivated, was made upon Carroll in his lodge. Three gardeners, who may also have been in Mr Farran's employment, named Kelly, Rooney and O'Donnell, conspired in the affair after, it was said, Carroll had lodged a complaint against Kelly, who in turn described Carroll as an 'Orangeman'. The *Freeman's Journal* of the following day reported:

> Yesterday morning, about two o'clock, a numerous banditti, said to be forty in number, attacked the country house of Charles Farren, Esq., which is situated near Rathmines Road, adjoining the avenue that leads to Rathfarnham Road. They first entered the gardener's lodge, in which was a poor man, in the service of Mr. Farren, named Daniel Carroll, who giving what resistance he could to the barbarians, they cruelly put him to death, and which we since understand was the chief purpose for which they came to that place.

The 'numerous banditti' was the basis of the story put about by the perpetrators to cover their tracks. The reports of the time indicate that after the foul deed, they plundered the wine cellar of the house (presumably in Mr Farran's absence) and 'carried off a quantity of liquor to their homes'. A crime of such magnitude must have created quite a stir in the entire south side of Dublin. The unfortunate misguided trio were tried, found guilty and publicly hanged at Terenure crossroads. The issue of the *Freeman's Journal* dated 1 November 1798 records:

> Yesterday were executed on Rathfarnham Road, at the entrance of the avenue leading to Rathgar and Rathmines, Kelly, Rooney, and

O'Donnell, who had been gardeners to gentlemen in that neigh-bourhood, and had perpetrated a most barbarous murder on a poor, inoffensive man, named Carroll, carter to Charles Farren, Esq.

The above malefactors were conducted from Kilmainham Jail along the Circular Road, and through Rathmines, to the place of execution by the High Sheriff of the County of Dublin, accompanied by troops of the Rathfarnham and Crumlin Cavalry. The peasantry who were spectators seemed to have no pity for them, and believed they were guilty, though these criminals denied the fact. The bloody shirt of poor Carroll, who had been murdered, was placed in front of the cart before them on the way to the place of execution. Just before they were turned off, Kelly and Rooney shook hands; the former appeared in much trepidation. After hanging the usual time, they were cut down and their bodies conveyed to Surgeons' Hall for dissection, consonant to the letter of the law.

The route of the gruesome procession was by way of Rathmines Road, Upper Rathmines, Highfield Road and past Rathgar House, the scene of the murder. Justice was administered in a harsh and uncompromising fashion in those days!

One year later Charles Farran wrote to his married daughter, Martha, in England under the date 28th May 1799:

> The Country seems rather quiet owing I believe to the exertions of Governmt in punishing those offenders Daily brought to Justice for their Attrocious Crimes. Scarce a day passes but one or two of those deluded Wretches are Executed or sent to the King of Prussia to serve in his armies. We are preparing to go this week to Rathgar as Governmt has granted us a Guard of a Serjt Corporal and twelve men wch are placed at the End of the Avenew at the red house opposite Tuckers wch will be a great Protection to the Neighbour-hood and has induced the Inhabitants to go and reside in the Country as usual so that I hope we shall enjoy peace and quiet as we formerly did.

The repercussions of the Rising of '98 were obviously still affect-ing the country, the entire episode and Mr Farran's comments only emphasizing the huge divide between the two traditions in Ireland in those times, a divide which was not religious in its origins.

Charles Farran died on Christmas Day, 1808 aged eighty-five years and was succeeded by his son Joseph, who, following the family legal tradition, was also Clerk of the Pleas in the Court of the Exchequer and a Freeman of the City of Dublin. Joseph Farran soon set about improving his property. In 1815 he took a lease of an additional eleven acres from the two major head-landlords in the area. One was the previously mentioned Redmond Morres, who later became known as Reymond Hervey de Montmorency, whilst the second, Rt Hon Lodge, had by that time acquired the title of Baron Frankfort (undoubtedly the originator of today's Frankfort Avenue). It is very likely that as part of these improvements Joseph Farran was responsible for the construction of a new house which we know today as 'Oakland'. He lived there until his death in June, 1852 at the age of ninety.

During this period the surviving ruins of Rathgar Castle were still very prominent in the neighbourhood, as they are recorded in the fine drawings in the National Library by Cecelia M. Campbell dated 1817.

Joseph Farran and his wife Ann had two sons, Charles Jnr and Joseph Jnr, and two daughters, Barbara and Louisa, and it is these two women who were responsible for designing and decorating the shell-house which lasted until well into the St Luke's era.

The shell-house took more than a quarter of a century to construct, the dates of commencement (1834) and completion (1861) being incorporated into the design as well as the initials of the two dedicated sisters—B.F. and L.F. The shells for the decoration were collected in Balbriggan and the design also included the Farran crest of a stag coming out of a crown. The Farran family sold the property at the end of 1853 after Joseph's death the previous year, but the two daughters moved to Georgeville (now No. 16) Highfield Road and continued to have access to enable their work on the shell-house to continue. They died in 1897 and 1898, each at the age of ninety-seven.

### Oakland

The new owner of Rathgar House was Henry Walker Todd, whose address is given as Fortescue Terrace, Rathmines. Mr Todd was a member of the family who had established the drapery firm of Todd

Burns in 1834 in partnership with Gilbert Burns, a nephew of the Scottish poet Robert. A major investor in the enterprise was Alexander Findlater, importer of wines and spirits.

Henry Todd joined with the Burns and Findlater dynasties and Mr Johnston of the well-known bakery to found the Mountjoy Brewery in 1852, whilst the Guinness family helped them to establish the Dublin and Glasgow Steam Packet Co. which later became famous as the Burns-Laird Line.

It was H. W. Todd who renamed his new residence 'Oakland', probably because by that time there were two other properties claiming the title 'Rathgar House'. Unfortunately, Mr Todd did not enjoy his residence in Rathgar for many years. He died about 1863 and by 1865 Oakland had been sold.

The next occupant, Hugh Brown JP, had come to Dublin from Keswick in Cumbria, England, and was the great-grandfather of Dr Alan Browne, who for some years was a visiting consultant gynaecologist to St Luke's Hospital. Hugh had been a buyer in Mr Todd's emporium in Mary Street and then decided to strike out on his own when he bought out a haberdashery shop called Underwood & Co. Business prospered and within a short time, in 1849, he joined forces with another Todd's buyer James Thomas and together the pair of them formed Brown Thomas & Co., which still thrives to-day as one of Dublin's most famous stores. Business prospered and when at the beginning of 1865 the trustees of the will of H. W. Todd put the house and 14 acres on the market he felt able to purchase. His address at the time is given as 63, Leinster Road. As he moved to Highfield Road (as it had now become known), Rathgar was described as 'one of the most prestigious and desirable places to live'.

Hugh and his wife Marianne had three sons—Vere Ward worked in the family business, Hugh Dunlop was a Baptist pastor in a church in Harcourt Street situated on a site which later contained Four Provinces House and the Irish Bakers' Union, whilst another son, Robert, became a medical GP and founded a clinic 'Maison de la Santé' in Charlemont Street. Hugh (Senior), who had been a member of the Select Vestry of Zion Church in Rathgar died suddenly on 4 March, 1882. His widow continued to live in Oakland for over ten years with her son Rev. Hugh Dunlop until she moved to Glengyle (now Stratford College) on Zion Road. Robert Browne (who had added an 'e' to the family name) also liked living in the neighbourhood and set up practice in Hopeton, a large house at 33 Terenure Road East, in the now well-developed village of Rathgar. He is commemorated by a very fine stained glass window in the chancel of Zion Church which was erected by his family and is inscribed 'To the Glory of God and in loving memory of Robert Browne MD of Hopeton, Rathgar who died Apl. 29th 1913'. Most interestingly the window and its design are dedicated to 'Luke the beloved Physician'. One of his two sons, Percival, who qualified as a solicitor was the father of Dr Alan Browne and thus the family involvement in Oakland and St Luke's has come full circle. During these years the Board of Brown Thomas & Co. regularly made charitable subscriptions to various Dublin hospitals. One may feel certain that Hugh Brown would approve of the use to which Oakland is put to-day.

When Marianne Brown finally moved to her newly-built house on Zion Road in 1893 the purchaser of Oakland was Charles Wisdom Hely of Linwood House, Sydney Parade.

Mr Hely was the head of the firm of Helys Printers and Stationers, 28 Dame Street and, as we shall see, a very wealthy man. He had ambitious plans for the development of Oakland into one of the finest properties in the southern suburbs of Dublin and set about his task without delay. The following year he bought from the trustees of H. W. Todd land on Orwell Park which obviously had not been sold to the Browns. This gave him a rear entrance which he enhanced with the fine pillars and wrought iron gates which are in magnificent condition to this day. His initials CWH and coat of arms are worked into the design of the gates and the same are to be seen on the red-brick gate lodge which he built nearby. Two years later in 1896 he acquired the land at Sunbury known as 'Ashgrove' which was leased to Mount Temple Lawn Tennis Club. One of the conditions of the lease was that Mr Hely and family would have access to the club via a private gateway from Oakland. One year

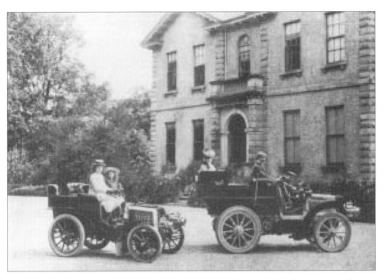

*Oakland in 1902: the extensions have not yet been added. The girl (aged 13) driving the second car is Violet Hely who, as Mrs O'Rorke, eventually sold the house and grounds to the Cancer Association Courtesy RIAC Archive)*

later he bought out his lease of Oakland, thus giving him freehold title over the entire property for the then enormous sum of £21,650. The landlord selling was a Thomas Pile who, only one year earlier, had bought the title from the heir of Hervey Francis de Montmorency, the son of Reymond, mentioned previously.

Charles W. Hely was also adventurous, and the arrival on the scene of the newly invented motor car soon attracted his attention. An issue of the weekly magazine *Motor News* in 1902 contains an article headed 'Mr. C. Wisdom Hely and His Motor Stud'. In it we learn that Mr Hely 'is as keen an enthusiast as one could hope to find'. He commenced motoring in 1901 on a 7 hp Panhard, of which he took delivery in London. Arriving in Dublin he 'was already an expert . . . and drove at a pace through traffic which terrified the onlookers and left the police aghast' (the car had a top speed of just 30 mph!). We can be re-assured, however, when we read that 'he has now covered between 5,000 and 10,000 miles without causing an accident of any description'. Within a few months he ordered a larger car, a 16 hp Napier and gave the little Panhard to his daughter Violet (who was to become the Mrs O'Rorke who sold Oakland to St Luke's). Although aged only thirteen Violet was apparently able to drive quite expertly. The magazine article concludes with this paragraph: 'Mr. Hely intends to use the car largely for running down to his fishing in the Mayo highlands. The distance is over 200 miles, and he expects to find it a comfortable day's journey'. Mr Hely did nothing by half measures and to facilitate the storage and maintenance of his cars he built a very large garage (called a motor house) just inside the present main gates on the right, where there is now a car park. This motor house had a turn-table built into the floor to allow for easy exit of the cars. The building survived for many years into the 1970s, having been used to store surplus materials left behind by St Luke's building contractors.

The next project of Hely was the enlargement of the house. The photograph taken in 1902 of his family and cars shows clearly (by its absence) that he was responsible for the building of the entire wing from the present board room leading down to the chief executive's office. He also built a billiard room (now the oratory) with a door leading from it out to a magnificent ballroom (also used as a theatre) measuring 120 ft by 50 ft and containing a small kitchen for catering. During this period the dining room (board room), the sitting room (library) and drawing room (clinical trials unit) were re-decorated with silk tapestry and painted ceilings by a specially commissioned Italian artist. Mr Hely had seven live-in servants, including a governess and a butler. In the grounds were a croquet lawn, tennis courts, a putting green, a rock garden and ponds. Traces of these features remain to this day. Four gardeners were employed to tend the grounds while the heated greenhouses provided a supply of fruit and vegetables for the house. In the early years of St Luke's an item in the annual accounts regularly recorded the receipt by the caterers of 'garden produce' to a nominal value of £200 p.a. One can visualize the gala balls, birthdays, garden parties and wedding receptions which must have made Oakland one of the centres of the Dublin social scene.

Charles W. Hely died on 31 December, 1929 and his wife Edith Mary continued in residence. In 1936 she sold the avenue (now

Oakland Drive) and land on each side to James Steward, a builder, of Fortfield House. The conveyance contains the condition: 'excluding the entrance gates and railings which are to be taken down and re-erected by the Lessors'. Thus the gates were moved from Highfield Road to their present location.

Mrs Hely survived until 18 September, 1944. Her daughter, Violet, had married Major Johnnie O'Rorke and on 21 September 1950 Violet Hutchinson O'Rorke closed the sale of the house and lands of Oakland to The Cancer Association of Ireland for £26,000. It included 3 lodges and various ground rents. The auctioneers' brochure stated that the property comprised 13½ acres to be sold with vacant possession and was held 'For Ever'.

The most exciting phase in the long history of Rathgar House and Oakland was about to commence.

### Acknowledgements

I wish to thank the following for their help in compiling this Appendix: Dr Alan Browne, Zion Road, Rathgar; Sarah Donaldson, National Gallery; Gabrielle Doyle, Oncology Resource Centre (Library) St Luke's Hospital; Rev. W. Gourley, Zion Parish Church, Rathgar; Bob Montgomery, Royal Irish Automobile Club Archive; Kathleen Rochford, St Luke's Hospital; and the staff of the Church of Ireland Representative Body Library, the Gilbert Library, the National Library of Ireland, the Registry of Deeds and Trinity College Map Library. A special thanks also to my daughter Maeve Kelly for her practical assistance in putting it all together.

### Sources

F. Elrington Ball *History of the County of Dublin Part II* 1903
*Census of Ireland* 1901
Suzanne Bloxham née Farran, letters
F. E. Dixon *The History of Rathgar* Dublin 1991
Alex Findlater *Findlaters—The Story of a Dublin Merchant Family* Dublin 2001
*Freeman's Journal* 1798
Weston St John Joyce *The Neighbourhood of Dublin* 1912

Deirdre Kelly *Four Roads to Dublin* Dublin 1995

Anne Haverty *Elegant Times—A Dublin Story* Dublin 1995

Pat Liddy *Dublin—A Celebration* Dublin 2000

Colm Lennon *The Lords of Dublin in the Age of Reformation* Dublin 1989

*Motor News* 1902

Angela O'Connell *The Rathmines Township* Dublin 1998

# Appendix 2: Board Members*

## 1. Cancer Association of Ireland Ltd

### 1950–55

*For five-year term from 29 June 1950 to 28 June 1955*

Mr George E. Russell, Chairman (Limerick)

Dr M.J. Brady

Mr T. J. Brady

Dr Oliver Chance

Mr F.C. King

Dr P. MacCarville

Prof. James M. O'Donovan (Cork)

Mr John O'Hanrahan, Surgeon (Roscommon)

Mr Matthew Russell, Surgeon

Mr Robert E. Whelan

Dr James Deeny from 1 June 1954

Mr Owen P. Hargadon from 1 June 1954

### 1955–9

*For five-year term from 29 June 1955 (Board disbanded in 1959)*

Mr George E. Russell, Chairman—resigned 12 February1959

Dr Patrick C. Bresnihan (Mayo)

Dr James A. Deeny—28 September 1958

Mr Justice William Shannon—resigned 5 February 1956

Dr John F. McEnerny—died January 1956

Mr Robert E. Whelan—resigned 29 July1957 at request of Minister

Mr Owen P. Hargadon

Dr John J. Kearney (Cork)

Prof. James M. O'Donovan (Cork)—resigned 12 February 1959

* The research for the bulk of this listing was done by Ethel McKenna
as Secretary to the Board.

Mr Terence de Vere White from 30 November 1956

Mr A.B. Clery, Surgeon, from 30 November 1956

Dr F. J. O'Donnell from 30 November 1956

Mr Richard W. Tunney from 20 December 1956—resigned 12 Feb
ruary 1959

Mr Christopher J. O'Reilly from 2 January 1957—filling vacancy

Mr H. M. Hughes from 2 January 1957—filling vacancy—died 18
January 1959

Mr Reginald P. Redmond from 17 December 1957

Dr Neans de Paor from 1 January 1958

Dr Malachy A. Powell from 5 November 1958—filling vacancy of
Dr James Deeny

Mr Owen P. Hargadon replaced George Russell as Chairman from
14 March 1959

20 May 1959—all members of the Board were requested by the Min
ister to resign their membership.

## 2 St Luke's Hospital Ltd

### 1960–4

*Reappointed for a five-year term from 20 May 1959*

Mr Owen P. Hargadon—Chairman

Prof. J. J. Kearney (Cork)—died during term

Dr Neans de Paor—died 27 December 1963

Mr Reginald. P. Redmond

Dr Malachy A. Powell

*Also appointed from 20 May 1959*

Senator Mrs Jane Dowdall (Cork) 20 May 1959

Prof. Denis J. O'Sullivan (Cork) from 22 April 1963 (filling vacancy
occasioned by the death of Prof. J. J. Kearney)

Mr John R. O'Mahony from 24 February 1964 (filling vacancy
occasioned by the death of Dr N. de Paor)

### 1964–8

*For four-year term from 20 May 1964*

Mr Owen P. Hargadon—Chairman

Mr Reginald P. Redmond

Dr Malachy A. Powell

# Board members

Mrs Jane Dowdall
Prof. Denis J. O'Sullivan
Mr John F. O'Mahony

### 1968–72

*For four-year term from 20 May 1968*
Mr Owen P. Hargadon—Chairman
Mr Reginald P. Redmond
Dr Malachy A. Powell
Mrs Jane Dowdall
Prof. Denis J. O'Sullivan
Mr John F. O'Mahony—resigned 19 March 1970

### 1972–6

*For four-year term from 20 May 1972*
Mr Owen P. Hargadon—Chairman
Mr Reginald P. Redmond
Dr Malachy A. Powell
Mrs Jane Dowdall—died on 10 December 1974
Prof. Denis J. O'Sullivan—resigned during term
Prof. Michael P. Brady (Cork) from 12 January 1976—replacing Prof.
    D. J. O'Sullivan

### 1976–80

*For four-year term from 20 May 1976*
Mr Owen P. Hargadon—Chairman
Mr Reginald P. Redmond
Dr Malachy A. Powell
Prof. Michael P. Brady—resigned 12 November 1979
Mr Liam J. P. Egan from 14 December 1976
Dr Bryan G. Alton from 14 December 1976
Senator Michael Mullen from 14 December 1976
Mr Noel Harris from 14 December 1976—resigned 8 September 1977
Dr E. V. Rutledge from 14 December 1976
Sr M. Columba McNamara from 25 October 1977 (replacing Mr
    Noel Harris)

### 1980–84

*From September 1980 for term ending 19 May 1984*

Mr Reginald P. Redmond—Chairman

Dr Bryan G. Alton

Sr M. Columba McNamara

Dr Malchy A. Powell

Mr Liam J.P. Egan

Mr Dermot O'Flynn

Prof. Ciaran McCarthy (Galway)

Mr Michael Doherty (Longford) from 30 June 1981

Mr Peter C. Murray from 24 February 1982

Mr Niall M. Hogan from 17 December 1982—replacing Mr Michael
     Mullen, deceased

### 1984–8

*From September 1984 for term ending 31 August 1988*

Mr Reginald P. Redmond—Chairman

Dr Bryan G. Alton

Prof. Ciaran McCarthy

Mr Dermot O'Flynn

Mr Liam J. P. Egan—died 24 March 1986

Dr Patrick A. Browne

Dr Niall Tierney

Dr Jane Buttimer

Mr Patrick Shanley

Sr M. Columba McNamara

Mr Brendan G. Doyle from 16 June 1986—replacing Mr L. J. P.
     Egan, deceased

### 3 St Luke's and St Anne's

*St Luke's and St Anne's Board (Establishment) Order 1988*

### 1988–92

*For four-year term from 19 December 1988*

Mr R. P. Redmond—Chairman for two years, then Vice-Chairman
     for two years

Mr T. Kevin O'Donnell—Chairman for two years

Dr John G. Cooney—Vice-Chairman for two years

# Board members

Dr Niall Tierney

Mr Patrick Shanley

Dr Bryan G. Alton—died 19 January 1991

Sr Laurentia Roche (Cork)

Sr Bernadette MacMahon

Sr Marie McKenna

Sr Catherine Mulligan

Mr George Eaton from 14 February 1992—did not take up
    appointment

## 1992–4

*For two-year term from 19 December 1992*

Mr Brian A. Slowey—Chairman

Mr Michael Doherty

Mr Derry O'Donovan

Mr Padraic A. White

Mr Donal O'Mahony

Dr John G. Cooney

Sr Bernadette MacMahon

Sr Marie McKenna

Sr Catherine Mulligan

Mr Kevin O'Donnell

## 1994–6

*From 19 December 1994 for term ending 31 December 1996*

Mr Brian Slowey—Chairman

Mr Frank Flannery

Mr Donal O'Mahony

Mr Paddy Shanley

Ms Norma Smurfit—did not take up appointment

Dr John G. Cooney

Mr Kevin O'Donnell

Sr Marie McKenna

Sr Catherine Mulligan

Sr Bernadette McMahon

Ms Kay Conroy—April 1995

Sr Antoinette Kelleher—September 1996

### 1997–8

*From 1 January 1997 for term ending 30 June 1998*

Mr Brian Slowey—Chairman
Mr Frank Flannery
Mr Donal O'Mahony
Mr Paddy Shanley
Dr John G. Cooney
Mr Kevin O'Donnell
Sr Catherine Mulligan
Sr Bernadette McMahon
Ms Kay Conroy
Sr Antoinette Kelleher

### 4. St Luke's Hospital

*Statutory Instrument 253 of 1999*

### 1999–2003

*From 22 December 1999 for term ending 22 December 2003*

Mr Padraic White—Chairman
Ms Claire Goddard—to March 2002
Ms Louise Richardson—from June 2000 to July 2002
Mr Barry Dempsey—resigned September 2002
Mr John McCormack—from October 2002
Dr Sheelagh Ryan
Dr Diarmuid O'Donoghue
Dr Claire McNicholas
Mr Derry O'Donovan
Mr Liam Dunbar
Ms Noirin Slattery
Mrs Mary Courtney

### 2003–7

*From 23 December 2003 for term ending 23 December 2007*
(Ministerial nominees unless otherwise specified)

Mr Padraic White—Chairman
Prof. Muiris FitzGerald—St Vincent's Hospital
Mr John McCormack—Irish Cancer Society
Dr Sheelagh Ryan—CEO Group

# Board members

Dr Claire McNicholas—Irish College of General Practitioners

Ms Jean Manahan—Irish Hospice Foundation—resigned June 2004

Prof. Diarmuid Shanley—resigned October 2005

Mr Chris Flood—resigned February 2006

Mr Derry O'Donovan

Ms Noirin Slattery

Mr Eugene Murray—Irish Hospice Foundation from September 2004

Prof. Dermot Kelleher—replacing Prof. Diarmuid Shanley from May 2007

Ms Gabriel Burke—replacing Mr Chris Flood from May 2007

# Appendix 3: Senior Staff

## Chief Executive

| | | |
|---|---|---|
| Liam J. P. Egan | Secretary-Registrar | 1952–74 |
| Esther Byrne | Secretary-Registrar | 1974–83 |
| Kathleen Rochford | Secretary-Registrar | 1983–87 |
| Robert Martin | Chief Executive | 1988–96 |
| Nicky Jermyn | Chief Executive | 1996–2001 |
| Lorcan Birthistle | Chief Executive | 2001–07 |

## Senior Medical

| | | |
|---|---|---|
| Oliver Chance | Medical Director | 1951–68 |
| | Rotating Chairmen | 1968–73 |
| Michael O'Halloran | Medical Director | 1973–88 |
| John Healy | Medical Director | 1988–92 |
| Michael Moriarty | Medical Director | 1992–6 |
| John Armstrong | Medical Director | 1996–2002 |
| Donal Hollywood | Medical Director | 2002–03 |
| Catriona O'Sullivan | Medical Director | 2003– |

## Matron/Director of Nursing

| | |
|---|---|
| Mary Dixon | 1951–79 |
| Margaret Johnston | 1979–85 |
| Nuala Duffy | 1985–94 |
| Eileen Maher | 1995– |

## Secretaries to Board

| | |
|---|---|
| Ethel McKenna | 1975–2001 |
| Marie Comiskey | 2001– |

# Appendix 4: Contributions by the Friends of Saint Luke's Hospital

Over the years since their foundation in 1980 the Friends of Saint Luke's have collected some €25 million. This represents more than one-third of the total capital expenditure of the hospital in that period. It is a noble achievement by thousands of devoted workers across the country. As a recognition of this achievement and a signification of the importance of this activity to the hospital, this list details the various projects on which the money raised, in literally hundreds of events every year, was actually spent.

1981–5
Simulator room
Simulator
Computer
Extension

1986
Radiotherapy Department extension
Diagnostic camera equipment
Simulator processor
Geriatric chairs

1987
Radiotherapy Department extension
Diagnostic camera equipment
Simulator processor
Geriatric chairs
Cobalt source

# A Haven in Rathgar—St. Luke's

Hospital beds
Infusion pumps
Clinics

1988
Image intensifier
Diagnostic camera equipment

1989
Linear accelerator
Hospital beds and lockers
Hitachi analyser

1990
Coulter analysis machine
Hospital beds
Canopy
Tannoy system
Automatic doors
Mini-bus ambulance
Seating

1991
Endoscopy system
Hospital beds
Fibre-optic system
Out-Patients' Department renovation

1992
Hospital furniture
Hospital beds
Water coolers
Seating

# Contribution by the Friends of St Luke's

1993
Phonyngoscope equipment
Micro selectron machine
Mould Room building
Seating
Drinks machine

1994
High dose after loading machine
Smoking-room renovation
Video system and scope equipment
Mound Room building
Syringe pumps
Nebuliser

1995
Aromatherapy equipment
Patients' hampers

1996
Mini-bus ambulance
Soft furnishing
Electric buggy
Oakland Lodge building and renovation

1997
Rehabilitation building including Activity Centre and physiotherapy
rooms
St Luke's Institute of Cancer Research annual grant

1998
St Luke's Institute of Cancer Research annual grant
Out-Patients' Department renovation
Carpets
Oakland Lodge patient information video

1999
St Luke's Institute of Cancer Research annual grant
Oakland Lodge extension
Christmas presents for children receiving radiotherapy treatment at Christmas

2000
St Luke's Institute of Cancer Research annual grant
Chapel renovation
Wheelchairs
Oakland Lodge phase 2 extension and renovation
Christmas presents for children receiving radiotherapy treatment at Christmas

2001
St Luke's Institute of Cancer Research annual grant
Oakland Lodge phase 2 extension and renovation
Audio-visual equipment for laboratories
Christmas presents for children receiving radiotherapy treatment at Christmas

2002
St Luke's Institute of Cancer Research annual grant
Christmas presents for children receiving radiotherapy treatment at Christmas

2003
St Luke's Institute of Cancer Research annual grant
Oakland Lodge phase 3 extension and renovation
Laboratory equipment
Christmas presents for children receiving radiotherapy treatment

2004
St Luke's Institute of Cancer Research annual grant
Oakland Lodge phase 3 extension and renovation

# Contribution by the Friends of St Luke's

Operating theatre renovation
CT simulator diagnostic machine
Patients' Christmas hampers
Christmas presents for children receiving radiotherapy treatment

2005
St Luke's Institute of Cancer Research annual grant
Oakland Lodge refurbishments
Patients' Christmas hampers
Christmas presents for children receiving radiotherapy treatment

2006
St Luke's Institute of Cancer Research annual grant
Replacement patient transport ambulance
Endoscopic washer
Colonoscope

2007
St Luke's Institute of Cancer Research annual grant
Landscaping of hospital grounds
CT simulator (pledge)
Patient Wellbeing Research Project

# Index

# Index